The Practice of Civil War Medicine and Surgery

In Historical Context

A Reference

Bruce Alan Evans, M.D.

ISBN 9798362631154
Imprint: Independently Published

Copyright© Bruce A. Evans, M.D.

Cover Illustration:

A ward in hospital at convalescent camp near Alexandria, Va.

Courtesy of the Library of Congress Prints and Photographs Division

Table of Contents

Introduction 1

Treatment of Medical Illnesses 3

    Apothecary Measures 5

    Principles of Medical Treatment 6

    Continued Fever 13

    (Alvine Fluxes) Diarrhea and Dysentery 20

    Intermittent Fever 30

    Measles 36

    Pneumonia 39

    Rheumatism 43

    Scurvy 46

    Smallpox 48

Surgical Treatment & Treatment of Complications 52

    Principles of Surgical Treatment 54

    Amputation 60

    Limb Conservation Surgery (Resection) 67

    Head Wounds 73

    Penetrating Chest Wounds 79

    Penetrating Abdominal Wounds 81

    Soft Tissue Wounds 83

    Probing Bullet Wounds 85

    Shot Fractures 90

    Erysipelas 92

Hemorrhage	95
Secondary Hemorrhage	97
Hospital Gangrene	102
Mortification of Wounds	106
Pyemia	108
Tetanus	109
Categorization of Medications by Action	111
Affecting Function	113
Affecting Function – Cathartics	114
Affecting Function – Emetics	116
Affecting Function – Diuretics	118
Affecting Function – Diaphoretics	119
Affecting Function – Expectorants	122
Stimulants – Astringents	123
Stimulants – Diffusible	126
Stimulants – Tonics	132
Sedatives – General	134
Sedatives – Depleting	136
Alteratives	140
Affecting Skin Structure for Local Effect	143
Antacids	148
Medications in the Pannier	149
Appendix: Glossary of Period Medical Terms	347
Author's Afterword	369

Introduction

A number of historical works on Civil War medicine have been published.

The focus of this work is somewhat different. The aim is to present the theory and practice of the Civil War physicians within their historical context. The information presented is almost completely drawn from period medical works available at the time and representing the "state of the art."

Once the poorly trained physicians were weeded out by rigorous examination and experience, Union and Confederate surgeons practiced high quality medicine for the times. It is instructive not to see that practice – anachronistically – as ignorant or mistaken from the viewpoint of the current knowledge of surgery and disease of more modern times. The knowledge of antisepsis, asepsis, germ theory, and indeed almost all disease mechanisms lay in their future. This resulted in empiricism, experience, and theory to shape available treatments. Their overall performance was excellent for the times.

One exception to this purely contemporary period presentation is the inclusion – clearly separated from the period information – of comments on the efficacy of the treatments from a modern point of view.

Sickness was as or more deadly to Civil War soldiers than were Minié Balls and cannon. Unlike previous works, considerable space is given to medical treatment and to each of the wide range of medications available, for each of which extensive period reference material is given.

Bruce A. Evans, M.D.

With regard to the surgical practice, detailed presentations of specific surgical procedure are not provided, but rather there is a focus on general approaches and principles.

Hopefully this work is of interest both to medical re-enactors and those interested in the history of medicine.

The Practice of Civil War Medicine and Surgery
Treatment of Medical Illnesses

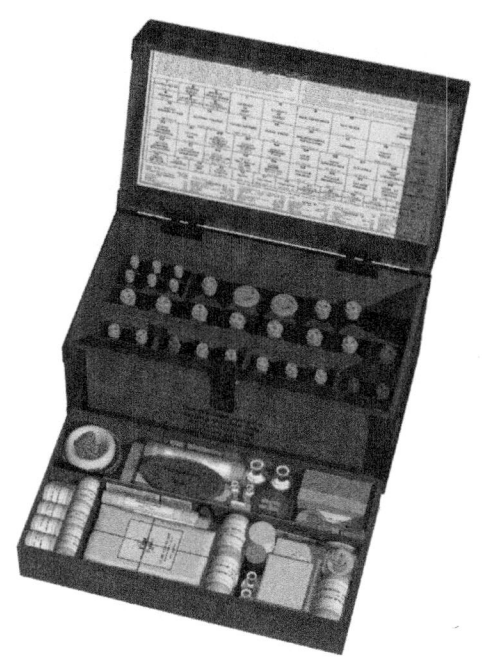

This section outlines the treatment of the most common medical illnesses facing the Civil War Surgeon. For each, the essentials of the diagnosis and treatment of the illness as directly abstracted from period medical text books are presented. Treatments are cross-referenced to the medications supplied in the Federal Army Medical Pannier pictured above, as representing the commonly available medications. Unfamiliar archaic terms may be understood by consulting the glossary in the appendix.

Following the historical context of the disease and its treatment, a modern perspective – set off in italics – is presented.

More information on the medications and their intended actions is given in subsequent sections on Medication Action and Pannier Medications.

The Practice of Civil War Medicine and Surgery

Apothecary Measures

Doses of the medications prescribed were usually given in apothecary measures, as below:

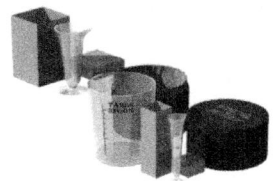

Measures (Apothecary)
Liquids:

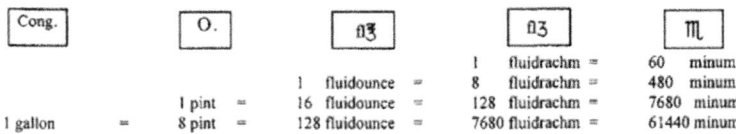

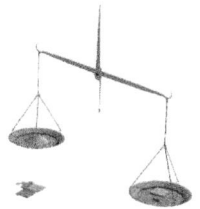

Measures (Apothecary)
Solids:

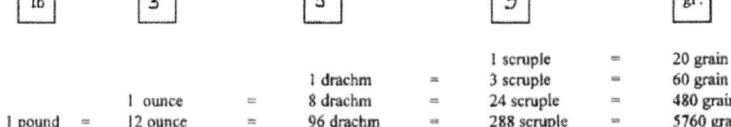

Principles of Medical Treatment

5

Bruce A. Evans, M.D.
Principles of Medical Treatment

Disease treatment has, as its goal, the return of the patient to the natural state. Generally, this is done through choosing treatments based on several different approaches:

Firstly, the symptoms of the disease often suggest that the deviation from normal is based on an excess or relative lack of nervous or vascular excitement in the involved tissues. Those characterized by excess - the sthenic diseases or phlegmasiae - show such signs as flushed skin, bounding and fast pulse, and redness, swelling, and pain of the involved parts. These are often best treated with the antiphlogistic treatments including a low diet and sedatives. In addition, causing increased tissue excitement in a distant or adjacent body area may serve to draw the excess vascular or nervous action from the diseased part, on the theory that the total tissue capacity for excitation is relatively fixed. This sort of revulsive treatment can be accomplished with medications that directly cause inflammation, for instance in the skin, or by medications stimulating body functions such as emetics, cathartics, diaphoretics, and so on. Those characterized by lack - the asthenic or putrid diseases - show paleness, weak pulse, a wasting constitution, and a low, muttering delirium. These are often best treated with a high, restorative diet, tonics, and stimulants. These theoretical treatments may need to be modified by experience - such considerations have led to the abandonment of bleeding for pneumonia, &c.

Secondly, some symptoms can be directly treated. Pain responds to anodynes. Tissue discharges, such as diarrhea or ureathral discharges, can be treated with astringents. The class of alterative drugs may benefit the symptoms as well, though the action is unknown.

Finally, for a few diseases, a true specific treatment is known, the use of which trumps the theoretical treatments above. The use of quinine for intermittent fever and colchicine for gout are prime examples.

Modern Perspective:

It is easy to hold both the treatments used by Civil War era physicians and the theories driving them in amused and horrified contempt from a modern viewpoint. We should, however, be both less anachronistic and more understanding. The science to develop treatments engineered to act on known physiologic processes was simply absent. Lacking that sort of treatment, the approach used made sense. Also, anyone who believes that even in modern times it is acceptable both to the physician and the patient to simply not treat if no proven effective treatment is known is mistaken. One need look no further than the use of antibiotics for probable viral "colds" and the wide use of "alternative" medicines — a surprising number of which were present in the pharmacopoeia of the nineteenth century — to verify that treatments of unproven worth are demanded and supplied. Hope, frustration, or anecdotal "successes" in previous experience may drive such treatment.

In 1861 medical knowledge was beginning to evolve from a mixture of theoretical "systems" of disease causality dictating theoretical treatments — often nonsensical to modern eyes — and a more practical empiricism that was somewhat less respectable academically. Lacking specific knowledge of most physiologic processes or any specific disease cause, symptoms became the focus of disease conception and treatment. The most prevalent theoretical systems in the United States contributed a number of "stimulating" and "depleting" treatments, the use of which was selected based on an judgement — based on whether the patient's symptoms suggested excess or lack of "excitement" in the tissues — of which type of treatment was likely to revert the constitution of the patient towards a normal state.

Balanced against these theoretical treatments was simple experience. This added useful tools to the theory-based treatments, including effective pain medicines such as morphine derivatives, anesthesia, smallpox vaccination, vegetables for scurvy, and quinine for "intermittent fever". Stark experience had by this point in time tempered many of the excesses of the theoretical treatments, as with the virtual abandonment of bleeding. The medical outlook of most well-trained physicians at this point was a product of the tension between these elements.

Advocates of experimentally based scientific medicine, led by the Paris school, were challenging this status quo. Specifically, many "heroic" depleting treatments such as violent purging were rejected. While both intellectually attractive and eventually productive, this approach had no actual improved treatments to offer at this time. Being seen therefore as essentially nihilistic by most practicing physicians who, after all, had patients who needed some treatment, the practical effects of the "numeric school" were limited to an erosion of the worst excesses of the theoretically based treatments.

Period Resource:
Modern Medical Therapeutics in the Nineteenth Century

Compiled from multiple sources.

A practicing physician's identity is intimately involved with therapeutic intervention, without which there is little reason for his existence. For this reason, many have little patience with the therapeutic nihilism of the Paris school, exposure to which led Dr. Wendell Holmes to produce his unfortunate statement to the effect that dumping all of our medicines into the sea would benefit our patients to the detriment of the fishes.

At the same time, the well-trained physician is not a mindless empiricist, trying to identify medicines that are effective for this or that specific situation by blind trial and error, like some savage medicine man, herbal practitioner, or quack who has no scientific concept of the causes of the deviations from the natural state we call disease. As physicians, we practice what might be termed a therapeutic rationalism. We use a conception or system of explaining disease that implies appropriate treatments. We do not relate a specific treatment to a specific "disease," but rather deduce what treatment the specific symptoms and circumstances of the patient imply with regard to a rationale explanation of the development of the entire disease state. Without this underlying understanding, we would in fact be the mindless pill-pushers we occasionally are accused of being by those who would profit by our denigration before the public.

Obviously, the theories of disease that guide our therapeutic choices have changed greatly over the years since the great Galen proposed the first widely accepted theory relating disease states to imbalance of the four bodily humours. With the passage of time and its consequent wealth of experience, and with the more recent addition of insight gained by the pathologic examination of diseased tissues, the theories underlying our activities become more perfect and exact.

The pathologic discovery of the role of vascular congestion in the process of inflammation has lent new weight, at least among American physicians, to the conceptions of Dr. John Brown. He described the "excitability" property of animals and man, and hypothesized than an imbalance of exciting or supporting stimuli may lead to disease states. These states can be roughly divided into the sthenic and asthenic diseases. This theory of disease has been very influential in North American medicine.

Sthenic diseases are characterized by excess excitability which leads indirectly to exhaustion of the tissues or the entire organism. Visible effects of this excess excitability may be flushing of the skin, increased force of the pulse, increased body temperature, vascular congestion at the site of disease, and so on. It is by these clinical characteristics that we recognize the sthenic diseases.

On the other hand, diseases caused by an insufficiency of excitability may be termed the asthenic diseases. These may be recognized by the inaction, and a times actual wasting, of the bodily actions or tissues. Signs may include a feeble pulse, bodily wasting, and great and early prostration of the patient leading to a quiet delirium in which the patient is poorly or unarousable, but lies fairly peacefully, muttering to himself. This stands in contrast to the raving, hyperactive delirium which might be seen in a sthenic disorder. The asthenic diseases are also often known as the low, adynamic, or putrid diseases.

It can easily be appreciated that this concept of disease directly implies the desired therapeutic actions needed in each case. Dr. Brown advocated increasing stimulus to the organism for the asthenic or low diseases. Examples of such action would include the use of tonics and a supportive or "high" diet. He also advocated decreasing stimulus for the sthenic disorders, such as the use of a scanty or "low" diet, and the avoidance of stimulating medications.

Further refinement to the theory has been provided by practitioners and teachers such as our countryman Dr. Benjamin Rush, who emphasized the role of capillary congestion with excess blood in the sthenic diseases, and Dr. Broussais, who pointed out the unique role of gastrointestinal inflammation revealed by pathologic studies of many of the sthenic diseases. These refinements led to the use of measures which decrease vital actions by direct effect, such as sedatives to heart action or the more subtle set of medicines which appear to reverse the inflammatory changes noted in the blood in sthenic diseases, such as the fibrin content or the thickness of the buffy coat of a settled blood sample. Although this rationale also provides a justification for the age-old practice of bleeding by venesection (in order to decrease the vascular force and excitement in sthenic diseases rather than to rid the body of "humours" as previously thought), this practice has unfortunate tendencies to cause severe prostration and an poor outcome, and has been replaced by more thoughtful use of local dry, and very occasionally wet, cupping for localized inflammation. Although we rightly reject the pathway of unthinking empiricism, only a fool does not learn from experience and modify his actions accordingly.

Perhaps more subtly, the practices of counter stimulation or conversion have been found useful, where production of an artificial inflammation (as the use of blistering agents locally, or in the process of revulsion, at a remote site) or the production of excitement in nearby but uninvolved organs by action of medicines (as with use of emetics or purging) serve to draw the excess tissue excitement away from the seat of disease. The treatments in modem use for the sthenic disorders may be termed the antiphlogistic or lowering treatments.

Additionally, we have learned that some patients who appear initially to be afflicted with a sthenic disease, will inevitably move into an adynamic stage of disease with subsequent prostration, and in these patients vigorous initial anti-phlogistic treatment will do more harm than good. An example of this type of problem may be seen in erysipelas.

Obviously, then, the division of disease states into purely sthenic and asthenic diseases is something of a oversimplification. Likewise, the division of medication action into purely stimulating or antiphlogistic (lowering) actions is a simplification. Some medications alter the quality of bodily functions, and this so-called alterative effect may be helpful in some disease states while not fitting precisely into the paradigm of effect on the overall level of stimulation of the system. Some of the actions of the mercurials, for example, fall into this category of therapeutics.

The art of medicine may be taken to be summarized by the principle of therapeutic specificity. This does not refer to a specific cure for all instances of a specific disease, which other than the use of quinine for intermittent fever, the use of mercurials for syphilis, and one or two others does not exist. Rather, therapeutic specificity refers to the physician's ability to tailor a treatment to the patient's:

Symptoms and findings, including but not limited to the determination as to whether stimulation or lowering treatment is implied

Character, constitution, and temperament, which will affect the extent of stimulation or lowering which will be necessary or tolerated

Geographic location, as regional differences in diseases, as well as in climate, affect the choices made. Southerner's exposure to heat causing decreased bile may mandate greater use of mercury, for instance, and bleeding that would benefit a northerner may injure the more phlegmatic southerner.

In the last several decades, there has been a general movement away from so-called heroic treatment of sthenic diseases, with copious bleeding and violent purging and emesis. Skeptics and opponents of modem medicine have suggested that this is due to a gradual recognition of errors in previous methods. More thoughtful analysis by the profession suggests that instead, in line with the principles enumerated above, there has been a gradual change in the distribution of disease manifestations, with more asthenic disease evident, and with sthenic disease now requiring, in the patients that we see, less drastic antiphlogistic therapeutic strategies.

From the above considerations, it can be appreciated that choosing a course of treatment and appropriate dosages based on the subtleties of the disease manifestations and the characteristics of the individual patient - the art of therapeutic specificity - is more important than the elucidation of a number of often artificially separated disease processes to the practice of the art of modem medicine. This flexible and learned approach stands in contrast to the ritualistic practices of the homeopaths, herbalists, and other so-called practitioners who the lapse of medical licensing laws in the last 30 years have allowed to pursue their doubtful practices on the American public. Rigorous examination of candidates for military medical positions by federal and state authorities are required to make certain that our troops are attended by physicians with proper experience and training in the true art and science of medicine.

Continued Fever

Unlike intermittent fevers, there are no clear remissions. The classic severe continue fever is typhoid fever, a putrid fever. A supportive diet is used, rather than a low, depletion diet used in many inflammatory diseases, due to the rapid transition to extreme prostration.

The onset is with feverishness, depressed spirits, muscular debility, and unusual relaxation of bowels. Additional symptoms next develop, including headache, back and extremity pain, aching bones and muscles, loss of appetite, increasing weakness and prostration, and typical rose rash spots on the chest and abdomen. Most exhibit a severe and prolonged course with 2-3 weeks of progressive symptoms, including, diarrhea, abdominal pain, restlessness, and somnolence with incoherent muttering at night. Recovery may follow, or complications may ensue, including pneumonia or, the most feared, severe abdominal pain with bowel rupture and death. If the disease is not fatal by the 5th week, symptoms may improve but the patient may die from extreme prostration. If patient recovers, convalescence is prolonged and tedious, and my be interrupted by diarrhea, pneumonia, and rheumatism.

Possible causes include fatigue, contaminated soil, food, or water.

Treatment of the sick includes a refrigerant diuretic such as potassium chlorate (Pannier #35), combined with tartar emetic (Pannier #5) if the stomach and bowels are quiet, or with opium (pannier #42) if these organs are irritated. Also useful are Spirit of Nitre (Pannier #12) if nervous symptoms are present and Dover's powders (Pannier #33) at bedtime for sleep.

Common continue fever is a febrile illness which does not run a typical typhoid course and is without other specific typhoid features. It usually resolves with perspiration or occasionally with gradual disappearance without prolonged tedious convalescence.

Modern Perspective:

Continued fever was a term broadly used to define those illnesses primarily characterized by a fever that did not exhibit the prominent and regular paroxysms of fever separated by periods of normality that characterized the intermittent fevers.

The most severe and dangerous continued fever was typhoid fever. This was recognized by many to be associated with compromised water supplies at the time. We know now that this disease is caused by a bacterium - salmonella typhii - that is spread primarily through fecal contamination. Many of the "public health" measures advocated to prevent or limit the spread of this disease were highly appropriate. The treatment of the illness itself - aimed mainly at the fever and the diarrhea - would have been largely ineffectual, aside from the use of opiates for pain.

Typhoid fever was separable from other continued fevers on clinical grounds at the time of the Civil War. Typhus, a different infectious disease spread by the Rickettsiae organism that was such a scourge during the Crimean War, was very rare. It was separated from typhoid by a different type of rash and the lack of the severe abdominal complaints associated with that disease.

Simple continued fevers, without specific features, may have been caused by a variety of bacteria or viruses, but were rarely fatal.

Period Resource:

Continued Fevers - Summarized from several medical sources

Unlike the case of the intermittent fevers, no clear remissions or asymptomatic interludes are present between the episodes of fever. The classic severe continued fever is typhoid fever. Lesser self-limited or less distinct although severe illnesses may be termed "common continued fever". Epidemic typhoid (typhus) fever, the scourge of the Crimean War, is exceedingly rare.

Common continued fever
This is a term for a febrile illness does not run a typical (for typhoid) prolonged course, does not have the typical "rose spots" skin eruption, when cerebral symptoms of delirium are not prominent, and when typical right iliac abdominal tenderness does not occur. In these cases the indefinite term is often used. It is also used for short duration illnesses that usually never come to the general hospitals, and are known by various other terms: simple continued fever, ephemeral fever, and irritative fever.

They usually begin with languor, lassitude, headache, inability to collect one's thoughts, restlessness or dream-filled sleep, constipation or diarrhea. Afterwards, a white-coated tongue develops, along with hot skin and a rapid and feeble pulse for 1-2 days. It usually resolves with perspiration or occasionally with gradual disappearance without prolonged tedious convalescence.

Typhoid fever
Typhoid fever is a typical low fever, adynamic illness, or putrid fever. The onset is with or without a chill, with feverishness, depressed spirits, muscular debility, and unusual relaxation of bowels. This phase might last days. Usually there are no episodes of perspiration. Then additional symptoms develop, including headache, back and extremity pain, aching bones and muscles, loss of appetite, and increasing weakness and prostration.

A few do not grow worse after 4-5 days, and recover in 14 days with relatively mild symptoms. Cerebral symptoms are limited to headache and restlessness. The typical rose rash spots on the chest and abdomen appear between 10-14 days, often visible very briefly.

Most, however, exhibit a more severe and prolonged course with 2-3 weeks of progressive symptoms, including:

-Active diarrhea, abdominal pain and tenderness, especially in the right iliac area, typanitic distention of the abdomen
-Increasing restlessness, incoherent muttering at night. Drowsy, dull, and stupid during the day, somnolent.
-Tongue: dry and dark tongue with deep red edges.
-Unconscious passing of stools; urinary incontinence or retention with abdominal distention and pain requiring catheterization.
·-Sordes gums and tongue

Recovery may be indicated by free perspiration together with a decrease of the other symptoms as the skin moistens, the tongue moistens and cleans, the mind clears, the appetite increases and a refreshing sleep occurs.

A variety of complications may prevent recovery and prolong the course:

Aggravated and prolonged diarrhea
Abdominal distention and pain
Intestinal hemorrhage with increased prostration (rupture of lymphoid ulcers)
Bowel rupture: Intestinal perforation (lymphoid ulcer) with exquisite pain, vomiting, hiccoughs, cold perspiration, collapse, and death.
Increased cough, chest pain, and hurried breathing with purulent sputum, bloody or rust colored, indicating development of pneumonia.

If a complication prolongs illness into 4th week, emaciation, pulse rapid and very weak, an extreme prostration occurs, and sudden death is possible due to heart stoppage. If the disease is not fatal by the 5th week, symptoms may improve but patient may die from extreme prostration. If patient recovers, convalescence is prolonged and tedious, and may be interrupted by diarrhea, pneumonia, and "rheumatism."

Typho-malarial fever
Also known as modified typhoid fever. It is characterized by distinct remissions with moist skin or frank perspirations which are not seen in typhoid fever. Recurrent chills followed by perspiration, especially if regular, suggest this diagnosis. The delirium is less frequent but more grave. Some feel the distinction from typhoid is important as "free use" of quinine would be indicated to deal with the "malarial element" suggested by the partially intermittent pattern of the fever.

Typhus
Typhus is thankfully quite rare during this war. Preliminary symptoms include malaise, back and extremity pain, nervous disturbance, and headache for several days. An abrupt chill occurs, followed by fever. The tongue becomes white, furred, and the face becomes dusky, livid and flushed. Constipation, scanty urine, and a shrunken abdomen develop. The disease then becomes asthenic, with a low delirium, and a dry tongue. Within 14 days the patient recovers or dies. The most specific finding is the rash - small red or purple livid raised spots, pinhead to one-half inch, appearing on day 6- 7, and lasting 10-12 days. As compared to typhoid, the duration of the disease is shorter, abdominal symptoms and diarrhea are absent, and the stupor is more pronounced early.

Prevention of Typhoid
To the extent possible, prevent:
- Over fatigue and sleep deprivation
- Exposure to excessive heat or chill
- Exposure to contaminated soil or "foul neighborhoods" such as the campground of and infected unit
- Use of tainted food
- Use of an impure water supply

Restriction of Spread of Typhoid
Remove the troops from the miasmic locale.
Locate a new water supply; until then use only boiled water (filtering

not effective).

Remove all infected cases to a hospital where all infectious material — waste, &c. — is controlled.

Extend the camp area to decrease crowding.

Construct new sinks; disinfect them daily.

Treatment of Typhoid

Irritating material must be removed, but with a gentle laxative only. Bleeding must not be done as it will worsen the prostration and collapse.

A refrigerant diuretic is recommended such as citrate of potassa as a neutral or effervescent mixture, combined with tarter emetic if the stomach and bowels quiet; or with opium if these organs are irritated. Also useful are Spirit of Nitre if nervous symptoms are present and Dover's powders at bedtime for sleep.

A sponge bath with water or alcohol plus water will help the feverishness.

For headache cold applications with or without leeches may be helpful; for abdominal pain and flatulent distention of abdomen dry cupping, emollient cataplasms, rubefacients or blisters to the abdomen are helpful.

For diarrhea: opium and ipecac, with or without acetate of lead or tannic acid

For nervous symptoms: sweet spirit of nitre, Hoffman's anodyne, camphor water or opiates.

For defective secretions, delirium, stupor, and abdominal distention use small doses of mercury to affect gums slightly, moisten the tongue, relax the skin, and decrease symptoms.

Turpentine is useful in advanced disease, when the tongue is dry and the pulse not strong: 10-15 drops every 3-4 hours for a day or two. Stimulants are a mainstay given the tendency to prostration and collapse: carbonate of ammonia and quinine in small doses may be used. If a collapse is imminent use powerful rubefacients in addition such as hot oil of turpentine, cayenne pepper in brandy, sinapisms, and blisters.

An appropriate diet should be supplied to the patients:

Week 1: liquid - rice water, barley water
Week 2: cereal preparations of gelatinous consistency; milk can be added later
Stage of prostration: animal broths, eggnog

(Alvine Fluxes) Diarrhea and Dysentery

The severity varies from acute diarrhea – simply frequent liquid stools – to diphtheritic dysentery with abdominal pain, tenesmus, and water stools mixed with mucous and tissue from the colon. Mild disease usually rapidly recover; more serious disease my resolve after up to 2 weeks, terminate fatally, or become chronic with gradual debilitation, wasting, and not infrequently death as the outcome. Diarrhea may often be prevented by proper attention to the sanitation of the troops, especially strenuous efforts to prevent fecal contamination of the water supply through careful placement of sinks (latrines) and prevention of flooding.

No universally effective, specific treatment exists. Mainstays of treatment are:

- A light diet recognizing the disordered digestion that accompanies the onset of the disease
- Initially, a purge to clean bowels of retained substances that may have begun the disease with Calomel (Pannier #41) and Rochelle Salts (Pannier #38)
- Some recommend use of an emetic such as Tartar Emetic (Pannier #5) at the onset; this use is decreasing
- A diaphoretic is used to increase sweating which may decrease inflammation and, some think, clean the blood: Dover's Powders (Pannier #33)
- Checking of flux with astringents through drying action on the bowels: Tannic Acid (Pannier #43), Lead Acetate (Pannier #51)
- Strength sustained with corroborants such as various tonics – Muriate of Iron (Pannier #50), Cinchona (Pannier #22) – and an appropriate supportive diet.

Modern Perspective:

These diseases were responsible for much of the misery brought by illness to the Civil War soldier.

Although the precise cause was unknown (see below) principles of sanitation that would help control these diseases were not, as can be seen from the digest of contemporary viewpoints. For a number of reasons, it proved difficult for the Medical Service to enforce appropriate location and use of latrines ("sinks") as well as standards of cleanliness that could minimize the impact of the diarrheas on the troops. These included ignorance and resistance on the part of the soldiers themselves, a lack of understanding of the importance of such measures on the part of the line officers, and the primitive conditions and often limited water supplies of the camp sites and march routes.

We now understand that the vast majority of these acute and chronic diarrheas are due to bacteria (such as E. Coli) and parasites (such as Entamoebae Histolytica and Giardia). Most of these are spread mainly through fecal contamination of food and water supplies. Spoiled food was another source of infection, although this source has a tendency to cause somewhat more self-limited diarrheal illness. Without any effective antimicrobial therapy, even had this been understood the treatments available would not have been effective. While opium products do exert some control over simple diarrhea, without some way to deal with the underlying infection, these products only control the symptoms imperfectly, and unless the disease is naturally self-limited - such as streptococcal "food poisoning" - do not cure. This was recognized. Only the natural resistances of the body were available to these soldiers to resist these infections. If they were already weakened by malnutrition and subclinical scurvy (referred to as the "scorbutic taint"), they were even more susceptible. The chronically undersupplied Confederate soldier was especially at risk.

The various strategies to "clean" the colon through early purging and to treat the suspected inflammation through revulsion - by causing irritation through induced vomiting or by inducing sweating - are ineffective. Mercury and antimony products were likewise ineffective but nowhere near as harmless. Also toxic was the primary astringent or drying agent used, lead acetate (which was still being recommended at the turn of the century by a very eminent Internist, Dr. William Osler, in his textbook).

On the other hand, the principles of dietary limitation to rest the GI tract were sound, given the inability to supplement these with intravenous fluids and nutrition and continuous gastric suction as might be used now, if necessary. The gradual wasting of the chronic cases could not be prevented without this sort of nutritional supplementation.

Period Resource:

Alvine Fluxes (diarrheas)- Abstracted from various medical sources:

Acute diarrhea
Diarrhea is simply frequent liquid stools without tenesmus.
The severity may be judged by the character of the stools, ranging from watery in secretory diarrhea to the presence of pus in inflammartory diarhea. More severe disease may be associated with dyspepsia. There may be griping abdominal pains relieved by bowel movements, with mild abdominal tenderness. The stool is usually feculent (containing obvious fecal matter), with a variable degree of wateriness, sometimes with scraps of food evident. The usual course is rapid improvement and return to natural state. Increasingly foul or

putrid stools may signal a progression to more serious disease. The usual pathology seen in specimens is normal bowel or simple inflammation without ulceration in the small intestine and some of colon, usually sparing the rectum and the adjacent colon.

Acute dysentery

When the patient complains of painful expulsive contractions (tenesmus) the distal colon and rectum have become involved in the pathologic process, and the more severe disease is termed dysentery. Simple inflammatory (catarrhal) dysentery is usually mild, self-limited in a matter of days and responds well to medication. The symptoms usually begin with griping abdominal pain (tormia) and painful expulsive efforts (tenesmus) resulting in watery stools, perhaps mixed with some mucous and blood. Obvious fecal matter disappears from the stools. Within 24 hours decreased appetite, nausea, and disturbed sleep occur and the patient may begin to decline. After 2-14 days the symptoms resolve, develop into the more severe diphtheritic form, or become chronic.

Diphtheritic dysentery occurs when the disease is severe and protracted. There is a higher likelihood of chronic or fatal outcome in this form of the disease, which may develop out of simple diarrhea, out of catarrhal form, as the fatal event in chronic flux, or occasionally, de novo. It may begin with chills and fever. Symptoms appear as above but intensified, and progress instead of resolving, leading progressively to debilitation, emaciation, "dysenteric collapse", cool extremities, sunken eyes, diffusely tender abdomen with occasional distention, vacant expression, muttering delirium or more likely simple unresponsiveness. The patient may develop strangury or vesicle tenesmus (thought to be due to rectal inflammation affecting the bladder neck as well as irritation due to the concentrated, scanty urine characteristic of the disease).

Stools reveal red or yellow morsels in serous discharge - like "meat bits in bloody water" - representing sloughed pseudo-membrane from the colon. This stool change precedes or accompanies the clinical deterioration. Preceding a fatal outcome, the stools become black and of "horrible" odor, and larger membrane fragments are discharged. Hiccoughs are a "universally bad sign." Improvement in stool, with development of feculent material present signals recovery. Convalescence is always tedious and tenuous, with relapses a frequent occurrence.

Chronic flux

When the diarrhea and any associated symptoms persist beyond a few weeks, the disease is termed chronic flux. In addition to the potential fatal outcomes referred to above, the patient may develop a liver abscess - signaled by pain in the area, and increasing liver size to percussion, and sometimes by a dry cough. This abscess may rupture into chest, abdomen, or bowel with fatal hemorrhaging resulting.

Treatment - Prevention

Diarrhea may often be prevented by proper attention to the surroundings of the troops. Every attention needs to be directed towards:

- Reducing crowding
- Finding the best water source for drinking, with strenuous efforts to prevent fecal contamination through careful placement of sinks and prevention of flooding
- Procurement of fresh vegetables in the diet to prevent a scorbutic element which predisposes to diarrhea
- Use of disinfectants in the sinks, &c.

For the hospitalized patients with flux, the flux patients must be separated from the others, and careful disposal of dejecta and soiled clothing will help prevent spread of the disease. No medication has been shown to prevent occurrence of the disease.

Treatment - General

Bed rest is helpful, in uncrowded wards. In general, cleanliness of surroundings and person promotes a good outcome.

Excellent ventilation is preferred, which suggests the use of tents or Pavilion-type hospitals rather than converted buildings for hospitals. Disinfectants need to be added to bedpans prior to use, and prompt disposal and personal washing undertaken after such use. The sinks for disposal of dejecta should also be treated with a disinfectant such as iron sulphate plus carbolic acid.

The Practice of Civil War Medicine and Surgery

Some surgeons have become aware of small organisms looking like yeast and others in normal stool when viewed with the microscope. The same is seen in stool of diarrhea patients. As no difference has been determined between the two, it is impossible to assign to these organisms a role in the cause of the disease.

Treatment - Diet

Digestion is greatly disordered in these diseases. Especially early in the course, only the simplest foods should be used. For water, rainwater or boiled or distilled water is preferred. Coffee and tea diluted without milk may be given. In general alcohol should be avoided, although in may be used later in the course of simple diarrhea alone.

For food, scanty food such as barley water and rice water is used. Milk, recommended by tradition, has been abandoned as it seems to worsen diarrhea. Later in the course, if patients are becoming wasted, boiled milk may be tried. Grain and cereal foods may be added after the acute phase, as should meat extracts, broth, and soups, all in moderation. When patients are improving, or in chronic phases, vegetables may be added. If a scorbutic element is suspected, fruit juices, potatoes, and onions should be used.

Treatment - Bleeding

The use of bleeding in various forms has a long history in the treatment of the fluxes. It has, however, been largely abandoned, despite theoretical claims of benefit by the action of depletion, when indications of active bowel inflammation exist, such as the presence of mucous and ejected pseudo-membrane in the stools.

Treatment - Internal medication

The general outlines of treatment have remained quite constant over the years:

- Initially, a purge to clean bowels of retained substances that may have begun the disease
- Some recommend use of an emetic at onset; this use is decreasing and not recommended
- Diaphoretics and Diuretics to clean blood by increasing

sweating and urination. The diuretics are now little used.
- Anodynes are used for pain
- Checking of flux with astringents through drying action on the bowels
- Strength sustained with corroborants such as various tonics and appropriate diet

Despite many fads, no specific, universally useful and effective medication has been demonstrated.

Purgatives

Saline Purges are frequently used as small doses of Rochelle salts or Epsom salts. Frequently used with rhubarb or senna.

Some use these agents after a thorough purge with calomel or blue mass. The majority, however, use only the salt.

Castor Oil, although nauseating, irritating, and often increasing the symptoms is nevertheless used extensively by some.

The use of mercury for dysentery began in India in 1700s, mainly for its antipholgistic effect rather than as a purgative. Overuse has led to much patient harm. Woodward suggests use only in a vigorous patient, only early in acute simple diarrhea or dysentery, and only in a dose of 30 gr. once or twice.

Hammond attempted to strike calomel from the Federal supply table in 1863 due to reported instances of toxic overuse, but a violent reaction from many surgeons prevented this. In summary purgative use:

1. Is useful to evacuate noxious matter accumulating due to decreased digestion and the fermentation and putrification resulting from the retention of matter in some areas of the bowels (at the onset of disease symptoms).
2. May increase secretion of intestinal mucosa, which is likely helpful. Some experiments indicate senna, castor oil, and rhubarb do not do this but increase peristalsis only; neutral salts do increase secretion, and "drastics" such as croton oil, colocynth do both but also produce direct inflammatory effects on the bowel, which likely should be avoided.

Emetics

The rationale for the use of emetics is that their action is revulsive for inflammatory colon lesions by drawing away inflammation to upper tract. Popular emetics include ipecac and tartar emetic, the latter often felt to have some additional, alterative effect on inflammatory disease. In general, emetic doses are out of favor, but small doses of tarter emetic given to increase sweating and for the alterative effect continue to be used.

Diaphoretics

Originally, sweating was felt to evacuate abnormal humors from body; a more modern rationale is that stimulation of sweating is useful for reducing internal inflammation through a revulsive mechanism. The effect is however not felt to be large. Dover's Powder (ipecac and opium) is the most common medication to achieve diaphoresis. The addition of opium to antimony in tartar emetic is for the same sweating effect.

Objections include the subject catching cold due to being wet, that the substances used have irritative effects within the colon, and that the effect in of minimal use in improving the disease course.

Opium

The main use of opium in alvine fluxes is as for the anodyne (pain relief) and soporific (for sleep) effects.

In dysentery, its use has been common from Galenic times to relieve pain of tenesmus and allow sleep. From the time of Sydenham to the 1860s, many physicians regarded opium as the most important treatment, often in large doses. A beneficial effect on the diarrhea itself, at least for the duration of treatment, has been observed often. There has always, however, been a significant opposition to such use. Early use in large doses does seem to bring bad results. It should be used cautiously, and only after the initial purging (due to inhibition of digestion and peristalsis by opium, which is thought to leave the irritating substances in the colon).

Opium products are often used in combination with other drugs such as astringents or ipecac Wood's textbook of Medicine recommends 5-10 gr. of Dover's Powder, but others have moderated this use. It is also used in chronic fluxes, despite the common observation that it "alleviated but did not cure."

Other anodynes are sometimes used:
- Hyoccyuamus especially combined with opium to increase hypnotic effect while decreasing constipation and digestive disturbance. (1/4 gr. Muriate of morphia with 2 gr. hyocyamus)
- Atropine
- Belladonna - suggested by some as specific for vesicle tenesmus and tormina; again, in combination with opium or morphia.
- Chloroform - given internally for tenesmus (20 minims). Repetition causes gastrointestinal irritation.

Astringents

Drying agents have been used since ancient times, especially for external use on ulcers, and other open wounds. This led to logical use in dysentery, usually as enemas but occasionally as by mouth. Their use is to suppress discharge and heal colonic ulcers. The vegetable astringents such as tannic acid have been largely supplanted by mineral astringents.

The most common in current use is acetate of lead, although careful attention to the total dose given over the course of the disease is necessary to prevent lead poisoning. Its use is a mainstay of treatment.

Tonics

Tonics are used in convalescence from acute dysentery and when progress is being made towards recovery in chronic flux.

Vegetable tonics such as Peruvian bark and quinine are heavily used. Small doses of strychnine have been used,

occasionally to excess, nearly as a "specific" for chronic flux. The antiparalytic action is seen as beneficial to the "paralysis" of the intestine that is felt to play an important role in advanced dysentery and chronic cases.

Other medications

Various applications are felt to be beneficial in some cases, mainly through a revulsive mechanism. Turpentine use is popular in this country. Wood has suggested its use for local stimulation and an alterative effect when the tongue becomes smooth and dry. His recommendation has led to frequent use of turpentine as a calefacient exciting warmth and as a drying agent. It is used by mouth and in enema, as well as flannel strips applied as a rubefacient to the abdominal wall for counter irritation. Sinapisms - mustard plasters — are used for similar reasons, and are appropriate mainly for mild diarrhea with griping pains. Blistering treatments are also used.

Intermittent Fever

Most are of the "simple intermittent" type. Paroxysms of fever occur every 2nd day in the "quotidian" form or every third day in the "tertian" form of the disease.

Paroxysms include:
- Cold phase: chills, rigors, lividity of lips and nails, nausea, and pain in epigastric, hepatic, or splenic areas. Associated headache and confusion is invariable present.
- Hot phase: fever, flush, increased rate and force of pulse.
- The paroxysm ends with a copious sweat, following which all symptoms resolve until the next paroxysm.

Frequent relapses sometimes long after apparent recovery are characteristic. Signs include an enlarged spleen, and sometimes diarrhea, dysentery, jaundice, debility, and anemia.

The mainstay of treatment in quinine (Pannier #34) repeated in doses of 3-5 gr. Or more every few hours during the remission. In addition, single large doses are usually given at the end of 1-, 2-, and 3-weeks following recovery to forestall relapse.

If quinine fails, Fowler's Solution (Potassium Arsenate) is used to prevent relapse. Treatment of associated symptoms includes Opium (Pannier #42) or Hoffman's anodyne (Pannier #20) for nausea caused by quinine, and Dover's Powders (Pannier #33) or opium (Pannier #42) with acetate of lead (Pannier #51) for diarrhea.

The cause is felt to be exposure to bad air, relating to rotting vegetable matter in swampy, warm climes.

Remittent Fevers wax and wane but do not have clear regular paroxysms with resolution of symptoms between. Treatment is with quinine, 5 gr. Or more 4-5 times per day, often combined with blue pill (Pannier#41) and opium (Pannier #42). The effect of quinine is less marked than with the true intermittent.

Modern Perspective:

The "simple intermittent fever" of the civil war surgeon was malaria, discovered since late in the 19th century to be due to a parasite spread by the mosquito.

Quinine, derived from the cinchona bark known to folk medicine in the New World for hundreds of years, is in fact a very specific and effective treatment for malaria, and is still used. This medication is one of the few specific and effective medications available to the civil war surgeon from a modern point of view.

Lacking knowledge of the specifics of the disease, and basing treatment decisions on symptom patterns alone, it is not surprising that quinine - so effective in intermittent fever - would be advocated whenever there was any suggestion of waxing and waning of the fever in other illnesses. So-called "typho-malarial fever" was one example of such a category. As a general medication for fever, or as a "tonic", cinchona bark and its derivative quinine were not effective.

Period Resource:

Intermittent Fevers — Compiled from Various Medical Sources

General
Intermittent or Malarial fevers make up 224 cases per 1000 reported diseases in Union army. They may be classified as:
I.   Simple intermittent fevers: paroxysms of fever and associated symptoms occurring regularly with symptom free intermissions.
II.   Remittent fevers: fever with periodic regular exacerbations with relative remissions but no symptom free true intermissions.
Most are of the "simple intermittent" type. Paroxysms occur every 2nd

day in the "quotidian" form or every third day in the "tertian" form of the disease. Frequent relapses sometimes long after apparent recovery are characteristic. Signs include an enlarged spleen, and sometimes diarrhea, dysentery, jaundice, debility and anemia.

Remittants

The onset of the disease is with malaise, then chills, followed by fever. Associated symptoms are many, including possibly:
- Anorexia, thirst, nausea, bilious vomiting
- Epigastric and hepatic tenderness, back and limb pain
- Hot dry and jaundiced skin
- Increased pulse, headache, tinnitus
- Delirium; constipation or diarrhea
- Coated, furred tongue

All the above symptoms wax and wane, often with regular exacerbations but no complete remissions. The disease often takes on an adynamic quality, with typhoid like aesthenia. The tongue cleaning signifies coming improvement; the tongue becoming dark presages deterioration with hiccoughs, low delirium, collapse, stupor, coma, and death.

Remittent Fever Treatment

The mainstay of treatment is quinine, 5 gr. or more 4-5 times per day, often combined with blue pill and opium. Frequently also used is calomel followed by a saline purge, but quinine treatment not delayed until results are obtained from the purge. Quinine is used throughout, but if remissions are well demarcated, larger doses are given during them to prevent subsequent exacerbations, with acetate of ammonia, spirit of nitre, and neutral mixture used during the fever periods.

For diarrhea, some physicians use turpentine. Dover's Powder may be used to "maintain bowels, promote perspiration, and secure rest." Iron persulphate enema is often used for GI hemorrhage. A few cases seem more "sthenic", i.e., "high" rather than asthenic, adynamic, or "low". For these, calomel or rhubarb followed by saline purges, a low diet, cold to the head, mustard to the feet (counter-irritant), and very rarely, bleeding may be resorted to.

True Intermittents

The patient may have preliminary symptoms including malaise, aching, loss of appetite, and nausea. The onset proper begins with a paroxysm:

1. Cold phase: chills, rigors, lividity of lips and nails, nausea, and pain in epigastric, hepatic or splenic areas. Associated headache and confusion is invariably present.
2. Hot phase: fever, flush, increased rate and force of pulse.
3. The paroxysm ends with a copious sweat, following which all symptoms resolve until the next paroxysm.

Intermittent Fever Treatment

Prior to cinchona, congestive aspects suggested bleeding as a primary treatment, but this was opposed by many due to the debilitated, "putrescent" character of the developed disease. In the early 1800s in India, bleeding and purging were used before cinchona treatment. In 1820, quinine was discovered, and the success of 30 gr. doses reported. Some continued to withhold quinine until "the portal and abdominal congestion and epigastric irritation relieved and febrile action moderated" by bleeding and purging, and then giving quinine during a remission. In the U.S., the use of quinine without evacuant treatment became the standard treatment as a "specific antidote to malarial poison." In Civil War hospitals, quinine is the sine qua non of treatment, although some use emetic and purge at the onset. The usual treatment:

Initially, quinine was repeated in doses of 3-5 gr. every few hours during the remission. If the paroxysms were so severe that worry over survival was present, the dose was pushed to the point of causing tinnitus, or given as a single large dose (up to 30 or more gr. at once) prior to the next paroxysm. Eventually single large doses supplanted multiple small doses for most patients. In addition, single large doses are usually given at the end of 1, 2 and 3 weeks following recovery to forestall relapse. If quinine fails, Fowler's solution is used to prevent relapse. For treatment of associated symptoms:

When called for by condition of tongue or bowels - blue pill and opium or, calomel followed by epsom salts, rochelle salts, or citrate of magnesia

Capsicum often given as adjuvant
If nausea or vomiting interferes with quinine treatment: opium, Hoffman's anodyne, ice, sinapisms locally applied
For diarrhea, Dover's powders or opium perhaps with acetate of lead or nitrate of silver

Pernicious Fevers
Congestive Intermittent Fever: a dangerous form characterized by the intensity and severity of the cold phase of the paroxysm. Often grave cerebral symptoms are prominent an early, including headache, drowsiness, coma, convulsions, delirium at onset, profound and prolonged collapse after paroxysm, and associated pulmonary congestion (seen in fatal cases). An associated intense jaundice is often seen in fatal cases, as is blood in the urine, and an associated hemorrhagic tendency. Pathology in congestive fever is notable for prominent petchiae (small areas of bleeding) and brain congestion without pus.
Treatment:
The mainstay of treatment is quinine pushed to symptoms of cinchonism (especially tinnitus) during the phase of collapse. Supplementary treatments used include mustard, emetics, capsicum, alcohol stimulants, stimulating enemas, hot frictions, sinapisms, and hot baths.

Chronic malarial poisoning
Malarial Cachexia:
The chronic disease usually occurs in those with a history of acute attacks, but occasionally not. This syndrome is characterized by:
1.   Anemia and an enlarged spleen
2.   A liver disorder with peculiar yellow skin but not actually jaundiced, as evidenced by the lack of discoloration of the conjunctivae (whites of the eyes).
3.   Anorexia (loss of appetite)
4.   Aches and pains, weakness, and tremors
5.   Occasionally edema, and even ascites (abdominal swelling due to fluid).

Treatment:
Quinine is used, but removal from the malarial environment often seems to be the only thing that helps.

Measles

This is largely a disease of new, unseasoned recruits, and is more common among those of rural origin. The disease begins about 10 days after exposure as a feverish cold (coryza) with photophobia (light painful to the eyes) and a cough within 24 hours. Then fever, headache, nausea, and possibly vomiting occur. On the 4th day there follows the appearance of small red papules (bumps, initially on the cheeks and forehead. Then, the skin lesions increase in size and spread to neck and chest. After 5-6 days, the symptoms begin to decrease (not coincident with the rash). As the rash heals by desquamation (loss of skin layer), the symptoms resolve. Complications that may prong the course of the disease include pneumonia, or less commonly coma and delirium signaling cerebro-spinal fever.

For a simple case the only necessary treatment is isolation and general support. For pneumonia counter irritants are applied to the chest and lower extremities such as brief applications of turpentine followed by warm applications and sinapisms (mustard or other irritant plaster), along with small doses of opium (pannier #42) and dry cups to the chest.

For diarrhea use saline cathartics such as tartrate of potassium and soda (Pannier #38) with rhubarb, then lead acetate (Pannier #51) and opium (Pannier #42).

Modern Perspective:

Measles - a viral disease mainly of childhood in modern times - could be a significant danger at the time of the Civil War. Many recruits were from relatively sparsely settled rural areas at a time when the nation, and especially the South, was largely rural. Without the exposure of their city-bred brethren, measles epidemics raged through the camps of new recruits. Deaths were caused by complicating pneumonia, or more rarely by a meningo-encephalitis - "brain fever".

It was recognized that no specific treatment existed (nor does yet). Once the troops were "seasoned", measles ceased to be a problem.

Period Resource:

Measles — Collected from Various Medical Sources

General

The fatality rate has been from 6-10%, usually secondary to the development of pneumonia.

The occurrence rate is about 30 out of 1000 troops annually except for the first year of the war, when the rate was closer to 70 per 1000. The decrease was due to the prior exposure of most of the susceptible individuals once the first year of the war was past (fewer new recruits).

Clinical

The disease begins about 10 days after exposure. Initially, the disease begins as a feverish cold (coryza), with photophobia (light painful to the eyes) and a cough within 24 hours. Then occur increasing fever, headache, nausea, and possibly vomiting. On the 4th day there follows the appearance of small red papules (bumps), initially on cheeks and forehead. Then, the skin lesions increase in size and spread to neck and chest. After 5-6 days, the symptoms begin to decrease (not coincident with appearance of rash). As the rash heals by desquamation (loss of skin layer), the symptoms resolve. A hemorrhagic form is sometimes seen, with an increasing intensity of the rash, petichial hemorrhaging from the mucous membranes, and consequent great constitutional depression and death. Other complications that may prolong the course of the disease include:

Most common: pneumonia

More rare: coma and delirium signaling cerebro-spinal fever
Treatment
For simple case: treat with isolation and general support
For cerebro-spinal fever:
1. Saline diuretics
2. Local cupping
3. Sinapisms to extremities and saline cathartics as a counter-irritant
For pneumonia:
1. Counter-irritants applied to the chest and lower extremities
2. Brief applications of turpentine followed by warm applications sinapisms
3. Small doses of opium
4. Dry cups to the chest
For diarrhea: saline cathartics with rhubarb, then astringents and opium.

Pneumonia

The disease begins with chills and fever, and an increased rate and force of the pulse. Associated findings include hot skin, flushed cheeks, headache, furred tongue, anorexia, thirst, and scanty urine. There is most often a thoracic pain, sharp or dull, a cough, and sputum streaked with blood or "rusty" in appearance. Labored, hurried, short respirations are invariably present. Examination findings include fullness to percussion over the chest and absent or "raw tubular" breath sounds on listening to the chest.

After 3-5 days, course may be resolution with decreased pain, eased breathing, and increased urine or progression to an adynamic phase, with rapid but weak pulse and a blackened tongue. In this case great prostration occurs, progressing to cold sweats, involuntary stools, muttering delirium, dusky skin, drowsiness, coma, and death.

Failure of the previously advanced antiphlogistic (especially bleeding, supplemented by depletion through cathartics, emetics, counter-stimulation, and a low diet) treatment of the acute phase of pneumonia has been recognized, and bleeding is no longer performed.

Therefore, this has reduced the acute phase treatment to supportive including purging at the onset with Epsom salt, compound cathartic pill (Pannier #31) or blue pill (Pannier #41).

The mainstay of treatment is tartar emetic (Pannier #5) early in the attack (1/16 -1/4 grain every 2-3 hours) with sweet spirit of nitre (Pannier #12) and morphine (Pannier #) a, with the treatment continued for several days. On the appearance of prostration, active treatment is necessary to support the patient and prevent final collapse and death. This includes a stimulating diet, using Beef essence, chicken broth, raw eggs, wine, sherry, porter, whiskey, brandy, and milk punch. Quinine (Pannier #34), compound tincture of cinchona (Pannier #22), citrate of iron and quinine, tincture of iron (Pannier #50) or other stimulants are given.

Modern Perspective:

Pneumonia is usually caused by a bacterial infection of the lung substance. The most common cause is Streptococcus Pneumonia, which is the target of the modern vaccination recommended for older patients more susceptible to the disease.

The description of the clinical course of the disease and the findings on examination, including those found when listening to the chest - stethoscopes were known and used, although they were simple wooden tubes put to one ear - are as accurate as may be found in modern texts. The disease occurred spontaneously, but was more likely to occur as a complication in a patient weakened by a wound or with other disease.

Lacking antibiotics, no specific and effective treatment was available. Given the excitement of the acute phase, with the agitation, flushed face, forceful and bounding pulse, rapid breathing, and so on it is not surprising that pneumonia was one of the last diseases to be treated widely with bleeding. By the time of the civil war, however, statistical studies from England and, especially, Paris were establishing the harmful effect of this treatment. Bleeding for pneumonia was definitely going out of style.

The other symptomatic treatments were, alas, largely ineffectual by modern standards.

Period Resource:

Pneumonia and other respiratory diseases
Derived from Various Medical Sources

General

The incidence of pneumonia is from 16-26 per 1000 troops annually. In 25% of the cases it is fatal, often in setting of a patient weakened through dysentery or continued fever. The disease begins with chills and fever, and an increased rate and force of the pulse. Associated findings include hot skin, flushed cheeks, headache, furred tongue, anorexia, thirst, and scanty urine. There is most often a thoracic pain, sharp or dull, a cough, and sputum streaked with blood or "rusty" in appearance. Labored, hurried, short respirations (30-40 or more each minute) are invariably present.

Examination findings include dullness to percussion over chest, absent or "raw tubular" breath sounds on listening to the chest, as well as moist rales (crackles) with breaths or friction rubs heard over the moving lung.

After 3-8 days, course may be:

1. Resolution with decreased pain, eased breathing, and increased urine. This is followed by a gradual normalization of the breath sounds over weeks (although occasional relapses occur).

2. Progression to an adynamic phase, with rapid but weak pulse and a blackened tongue. Great prostration occurs, progressing to cold sweats, involuntary stools, muttering delirium, dusky skin, drowsiness, coma, and death.

Treatment - early phase

Failure of the previously advanced antiphlogisitic treatment of the acute phase of pneumonia has been recognized, with a tendency of the patient to fall into an asthenic state of collapse. Bleeding is therefore no longer performed. Therefore, this has reduced the acute phase treatment to supportive:

Purging at the onset with Epsom salt, compound cathartic pill or blue pill. Neutral salines such as citrate or nitrate of potash may be used.

Veratrum Viride or rarely digitalis may be used to decrease the pulse

The mainstay of treatment is tartar emetic early in the attack (1/16 -1/4 grain every 2-3 hours) with sweet spirit of nitre and morphine, with the treatment continued for several days.

If no response is seen to this regimen, mercurial treatment is usually used to "decrease fever, allay inflammation, and promote resorption of consolidated lung tissue:" Blue pill and opium, calomel and opium, or calomel and Dover's Powder are used for this purpose, sometimes together with nitre and ipecac. Small doses are used, short of those causing constitutional manifestations such as salivation.

General "depletion" is, as mentioned above, rarely employed. For chest symptoms hot fomentations or dry cups may be used.

Treatment - adynamic phase

With the appearance of adynamia, the signs of which are mentioned above, active treatment is necessary to support the patient and prevent final collapse and death.

The best nourishment available for a stimulating diet is used, including beef essence, chicken broth, raw eggs, wine, sherry, porter, whiskey, brandy, and milk punch.

Quinine, compound tincture of cinchona, citrate of iron and quinine, tincture of iron, or other stimulants are given.

Blisters to the chest are used to promote absorption of the lung consolidation by drawing inflammation to the skin.

With a persistent cough, the addition of expectorants is undertaken, such as syrup of ipecac and squill, compound syrup of squill, or compound licorice mixture.

If the cough, expectoration, and intercurrent fever indicated the presence of a secondary inflammation, this should be vigorously treated with tartar emetic again, plus counter-irritants including sinapisms, turpentine stupes, pitch, croton oil, and cantherides used as local applications.

Bronchitis

Persistent cough without the evidence of the consolidation of lung tissue associated with pneumonia indicates bronchitis. This is generally treated with Dover's Powders, Spirit of Nitre, Neutral Mixture, and Ipecac.

Rheumatism

The cause of acute rheumatism is unknown, but it is perhaps related to exposure to cold and damp. The disease onset is with the sudden appearance of fever associated with pain and often inflammation of major joints. This may be associated with endocarditis (inflammation of heart valves).

For fever at the onset of acute rheumatism, often the use of quinine (Pannier #34) is appropriate. For internal use, most often the choices are capsicum (Pannier #1) and iodide of potassium (Pannier #37) or extract of colchicum (Pannier #48). This latter does not work as invariably for this disorder as it does for gout. Some physicians advocate a purge at onset – using calomel (Pannier #41) by mercury advocates or saline purges such as Epsom salts or Rochelle salts (Pannier #38) by others – as well as subsequent use of calomel for the alterative effect.

Opium (Pannier #42), laudanum (Pannier #22), or night time Dover's Powders (Pannier #33) are used for pain. External (local) treatment includes cupping to the spine, small blisters to the involved joints, painting the involved joints with tincture of iodine, cupping of joints, or application of cotton wraps covered by oiled silk or flax seed poultices to the painful joints.

Chronic rheumatism refers to painful, stiff, and tumid joints without fever. The term is generally and often imprecisely applied to "all obscure and painful afflictions of the locomotor apparatus". Due to the subjective symptoms many of these cases represent malingering. Treatment includes opium (Pannier #42), laudanum (Pannier #22), or night time Dover's Powder (Pannier #33)for pain; internal use of colchicum (Pannier #48) and iodide of potassium (Pannier #37), as well as local treatment of involved areas as for acute rheumatism. Results of treatment are poor and many patients und up discharged due to continued symptoms.

Modern Perspective:

Acute rheumatism was the term used to describe the sudden, severe inflammation of one or more major joints of the body.

In modern terms, this can have several causes.

Given the age of the usual soldier, many of these probably represented the Rheumatic Fever that can follow Streptococcal infections such as tonsillitis. We now know that this is a disordered immune reaction triggered by that infection which attracts joints and, frequently, heart valves. This latter association was also noted by the civil war era medical profession. Modern treatment is prevention by antibiotic treatment of the initial infection, and anti-inflammatory treatment of the disease with drugs that suppress the immune response. None of this was available to the civil war surgeon. Colchicine, which was so effective for gout - also a disease characterized by sudden and painful inflammation of one or more joints, although caused by a completely different mechanism relating to deposition of uric acid crystals in the joints - was by extension tried in acute rheumatism. It happens that colchicine does possess some general anti-inflammatory effect on the order of ibuprofen, so it may have been of some benefit, if not of the almost magic variety seen in gout.

Other causes of acute arthritis would be Rheumatoid arthritis, which can be seen in younger patients, and acute arthritis cause by bacterial infections. The former could spontaneously remit, the latter would progress to sepsis and death.

Extension of the term "rheumatism" to chronic joint complaints robbed the term of what specificity it had with regard to treatment strategies. Chronic rheumatism strictly applied would cover all the causes of chronic arthritic complaints, and more loosely applied covered many chronic pain complaints, including low back pain of uncertain cause. Musculoskeletal pain in a group of young men performing great efforts of exertion are not unexpected; nor is the ability of soldiers to describe such pain to be relieved from duty. Many surgeons believed that "chronic rheumatism" was a synonym for malingering.

Scurvy

The first symptoms of scurvy are tiredness, fatigue, and dull aching pains in legs and feet. At this point the symptoms are rather non-specific, and the diagnosis is rarely made. Stamina is, however, already decreased. Increased pain develops, typically involving the legs and back. This pain may be falsely ascribed to rheumatism.

Finally, more specific changes occur and the diagnosis cannot be missed: the gums become swollen and tumid, red, spongy and disposed to bleed. The teeth become loose and the breath offensive. Petechial spots appear, earliest of the calves and then more widespread. Then larger hemorrhagic discolorations appear on the skin, and edema of limbs develops that pits with finger pressure. Skin becomes dray and rough, the complexion anemic, pale, and waxy. The patient becomes debilitated and depressed. Any wounds are slow to heal; in fact, recent healed wounds may re-open. With continued and more severe disease, swollen gums become dark. Initially they swell sufficiently to cover the sides of the teeth, then tissue breakdown occurs with exposure of the roots of the teeth. Death my occur from diarrhea, pulmonary edema, or coma.

The disease can be both prevented and treated with a proper diet. Fresh vegetables (although some question their efficacy), fresh meat, and vinegar are helpful. Rapid improvement is usually seen with such treatment. Acetic, citric, and tartaric acids, salts of potash (especially bicarbonates (Pannier #36) and tincture of ferric chloride (Pannier #50) – 15-20 drops three times per day – are used as supplements. Without the proper diet, however, improvement will not occur.

Modern Perspective:

It had been demonstrated well before the 1860s that scurvy was a disease of dietary deficiency, and could be prevented through the use of citrus fruit juice - hence the name "limeys" for British sailors.

At the time of the Civil War, although the beneficial effect of a "good diet" were clearly known, neither the active ingredient - much later identified as what we now know as Vitamin C - nor which foods are especially rich in that substance was known.

Vitamin C is destroyed by thorough cooking. The foods which the surgeons were particularly interested in for the soldiers were onions, potatoes, fresh meat, and fresh vegetables. In fact, fresh meat, aside from the liver, has little vitamin C. Potatoes have some but are not an especially rich source, while onions have more. Fresh vegetables are the best source aside from citrus fruits, but were rarely available. Vinegar, also felt to be of use, really has no vitamin C, but can be used to preserve cabbage and other vegetables (sauerkraut) to prolong their "shelf life" and make them more available to the soldiers in the field. The infamous Union army desiccated vegetables, containing dried cabbage (rich source of vitamin C), carrots (almost none), turnips (some vitamin C), parsnips (some), and onions (more, but not a rich source) formed into bricks for storage and shipping was meant to address this problem. Unfortunately, the soldiers hated the "desecrated" vegetables and refused to eat them; the problem was likely compounded by unscrupulous contractors whose dried vegetables seemed to contain an unhealthy amount of stems and grass.

Smallpox

This devastating disease must be prevented. Military regulations mandate vaccination of all troops; unfortunately, many state do not take sufficient care that this is done. Further complicating prevention, many vaccinations to not "take", perhaps due to poor quality or inactive material. Therefore, only routine re-vaccination will identify those with an ineffective initial attempt, as they will react to the re-vaccination with redness, swelling, and crust formation. The disease is extremely contagious and begins 7-12 days after the exposure with repeated chills occurring over 24 hours, with intense headache, and back, leg and arm pain. Vomiting and nausea often occur. Fever, a rapid pulse, and occasionally delirium are early symptoms. On the fourth day the typical small red spots appear on forehead and wrists, spreading over the face and extremities. The temperature falls as the lesions mature, becoming pustules associated with swelling and redness. Fever, which usually disappears with the appearance of the rash, now recurs. The swelling, especially of the face and mouth/throat, may be sever enough to close the eyes and make swallowing or even breathing difficult. The fever and prostration continue, with increased thirst, swollen lymph glands, and delirium sometimes progressing to death in severe cases.

In mild cases, treatment begins with protection of the skin from damage. Laxatives, saline sudorifics – tartrate of soda and potassium (Pannier #38), and Dover's Powder (Pannier #33) are used during the fever. Tonics, stimulants, and concentrated nourishment are used after the fall of the secondary fever. External applications of creosote (Pannier #46) in olive oil (Pannier #25) or iodine (Pannier #4) in glycerin (Pannier #27) are used to decrease irritation and subsequent scarring. For mouth, tongue, and internal throat lesions acetate of lead

(Pannier #51) for the astringent effect and morphia (Pannier #39) for pain are helpful.

Modern Perspective:

*Smallpox is a viral illness without a truly effective treatment. Prevention is the key, and for hundreds of years vaccination with infectious material from the related but usually mild illness caused by the Vaccinia virus (hence the name "vaccination") has been known to confer immunity. Even before this was widely available, it was known that inoculation with infectious substances from a **smallpox** case usually caused a much milder form of the disease than that contracted "naturally" and conferred life-long immunity. So terrifying was this disease that many took that risk prior to the wide availability of vaccinia-based immunization.*

The substances used for vaccination were dried crusts from healing vaccinia lesions obtained from children or cow udders. This substance was not uniformly active, and therefore soldiers could be "vaccinated" and remain unprotected. Routine re-vaccination became standard.

The treatments for the sick patient were largely ineffective, other than for some degree of soothing of the skin and, when appropriate, pain relief with opiates.

Period Resource

Small-Pox — Summarized from Various Medical Sources

Preventative
The occurrence is 5.5 per 1000 troops annually with a death rate 1.95 per 1000 troops.
The lack of serious outbreaks is mainly due to a successful vaccination program. Military regulations mandate vaccination; many state military authorities unfortunately do not follow through, usually due to failure

to appreciate that a previous vaccination attempt does not take away the need for re-vaccination.

Successful revaccination implies clinical evidence of vaccinia infection such as mild fever, and not just formation of an appropriate crust at the vaccination site. As some vaccination material has been found to be inert, it is necessary to insist on this evidence of Vaccinia infection to be sure of the success of the vaccination attempt. The presence of some inert vaccination material has led to the practice of many physicians of rubbing together 2 or 3 separate crusts to obtain vaccination material. Crusts (and serum) are obtained for vaccination in one of two ways:

1. "Humanized" - raised and propagated through inoculation of infants in northern cities
2. "Bovine" - raised and propagated in cows (udders)

The reaction of troops to revaccination is used to estimate proportion at risk for small pox infection. In some supposedly protected troops all were revaccinated, and one fourth had a reaction (fever, etc.) that indicated successful revaccination, and therefore that number had been unprotected from infection regardless of the previous vaccination status.

Clinical

Onset of the disease begins 7-12 days after the exposure.

Initial phase: Repeated chills occur over 24 hours, with intense headache, and characteristic severe lumbar and extremity pains. Vomiting and nausea often occur. Early on, increased temperature occurs, with rapid and full pulse, and sometimes delirium. The patient becomes restless and distressed, with the skin hot and dry.

Eruption: About day 4, the appearance of small red spots on forehead (especially at the hairline) and wrists, spreading over the face and extremities is noted. The trunk is affected least and last. The temperature falls as the lesions mature, initially becoming raised with a central depression (umbilication), then becoming pustules (pus filled) associated with swelling and redness. The generalized symptoms and fever, which usually disappear with the appearance of the rash, now recur (secondary fever). The swelling, especially of the face and mouth/throat, may be severe enough to close the eyes and make swallowing or even breathing difficult.

Mild cases show discrete (separated) skin lesions. They have a gradually decreasing fever over 1-2 days, and then recovery with pus discharge, scab formation, and healing of the lesions.

Severe cases show many lesions becoming confluent (continuous) so as to form large areas of "superficial ulcer" over the face.

The fever and prostration continue, with increased thirst, swollen lymph glands, and delirium progressing to death.

Treatment

Mild cases:

Protect from damage to skin

Use laxatives, saline sudorifics, and Dover's Powder during pyrexia (stage of fever). Use tonics, stimulants, and concentrated nourishment after the fall of the secondary fever.

External applications are used to decrease irritation and subsequent scarring with cooling or astringent ointments. Applications include creosote in olive oil and iodine in glycerine.

Some paint silver nitrate on the lesions.

For mouth, tongue, and internal throat lesions, a gargle such as 30 grains of chlorate of potash in 4 oz. water, or chlorinated soda (1 and one-half drachm in 8-oz. water) are used. Also helpful is acetate of lead for the astringent effect and morphia for pain.

Surgical Treatment & Treatment of Complications

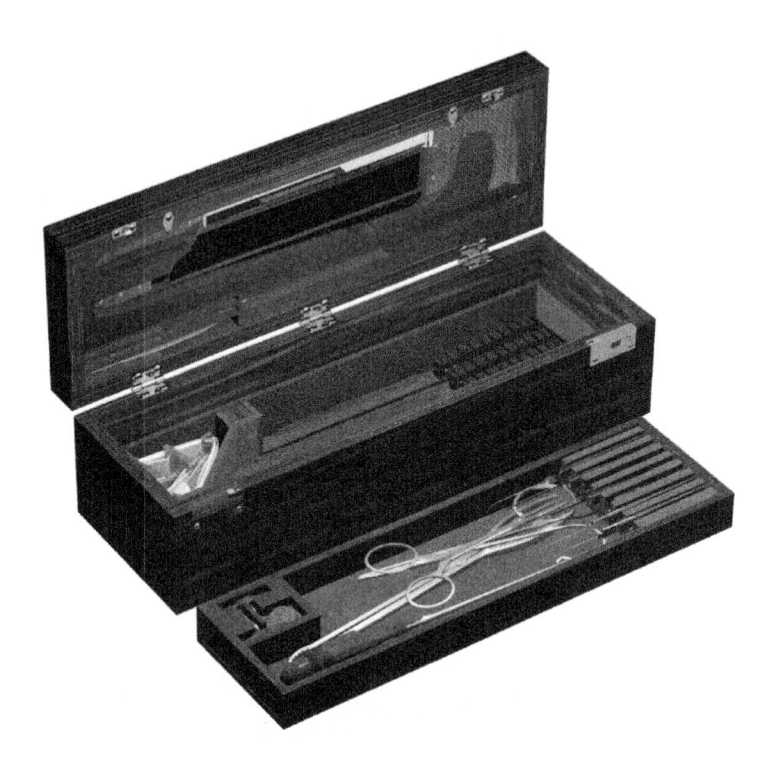

This section outlines the treatment of the most common surgical issues facing the Civil War Surgeon. For each, the essentials of the diagnosis and treatment of the wound or complication as directly abstracted from period surgical text books is presented. Drug treatments are cross-referenced to the medications supplied in the Federal Army Medical Pannier. Unfamiliar archaic terms may be understood by consulting the glossary in the appendix.

The Practice of Civil War Medicine and Surgery

Following the historical context of the wound or disease and its treatment, a modern perspective – set off in italics – is presented.

More information on the medications referenced and their intended actions is given in subsequent sections on Medication Action and Pannier Medications.

Bruce A. Evans, M.D.
Principles of Surgical Treatment

The initial job of the surgeon, when confronted with a gunshot or fragment wound, once any hemorrhage is controlled, is a careful examination of the wound. This must not be put off, for once reaction sets in with swelling, pain, and inflammation, the examination including the identification of missile tracks becomes impossible.

The object of the examination is twofold. Firstly, a judgement must be made as to the damage that has been done, and whether, for an extremity wound, the limb must be sacrificed to life. The existence of any fracture, especially involving a joint, must be determined for this purpose. Damage to blood vessels must be determined, and appropriate ligatures placed to control hemorrhage that may have been controlled with pressure or tourniquets until this time. For trunk wounds, a determination as to whether the lung or the abdominal cavity has been entered is made, although this tells us mostly if the patient will live rather than directing a surgical procedure.

Secondly, all foreign bodies in the wound that can be identified must be removed if healing is to occur. This includes retained missiles, pieces of clothing pushed into the wound, and fragments of bone.

The purpose of surgical treatment is to improve the likelihood of survival of a patient with a wound, and in addition, if possible, to minimize the disability caused by the wound. The initial treatment involves control of hemorrhage and careful examination of the wound before the stage of reaction with swelling, pain, and inflammation makes such examination impossible. Anesthesia is used for all such examinations if necessary, and for all surgery.

Soft tissue wounds, if not extensive, are best treated by removal of all foreign objects in the wound to prevent chronic discharge and failed healing, moist dressings, and appropriate medical treatment based on the degree of inflammation present on the one hand (mandating antiphlogistic or depletion treatment) and the degree of depression of the system on the other (mandating stimulation and supportive treatment).

Modern Perspective:

The two most visible effects of the bullet wound were the inflammatory reaction that inevitably set in by 24-48 hours and the drainage of pus that always occurred from the wound.

Over time, all of the available antiphlogistic remedies, both by mouth and in local applications had been tried, without much benefit. Depleting diets were found to be harmful despite the very visible evidence of inflammation caused, as we now know, by the ubiquitous infection.

It is likely fortunate that surgeons of both sides depended mainly on the water dressing for gunshot wounds. While not especially beneficial, neither was it particularly harmful compared to the alternatives, and the soldiers certainly seemed to find it soothing.

The coming of effective anesthesia made surgery practical and robbed it of much of its horrors. The period between the availability of anesthesia and the discovery and spread of antiseptic surgical technique was about 25 years: unfortunately for the wounded soldier, this included the period of the Civil War.

Most of the surgical strategy of the Civil War Surgeon for improving the chances for survival of the wounded can today be seen as logical consequences of the likelihood of life-threatening infections. Thus, soft tissue wounds usually heal if foreign bodies are removed. Extremity wounds without joint damage, massive soft tissue or blood vessel destruction, or severe damage to bone have a good chance to heal. Extremity wounds not meeting these conditions more often led to fatal outcome secondary to infection than did amputation. Hence, in these pre-antibiotic and pre-antiseptic surgery era, removal of a disposable body part to increase the odds of survival made sense.

Penetrating wounds of the head, chest, and abdomen were another matter entirely. These often-fatal wounds, for which contemporary surgical treatment had generally been found at best ineffective and frequently harmful, have several factors in common from a modern perspective. In some cases, death resulted directly from vital structures either not repairable or amenable to sacrifice (the brain, large arteries of the chest, abdomen, or pelvis) or inaccessible without predictable fatal infection (blood vessels within the brain, chest, and abdomen causing hemorrhage). In many cases they involve violation of sterile body cavities, with inevitable infection only worsened by additional surgical violation. Death resulted in these cases from the effects of that infection, either through a slow wearing down of the patient, involvement of vital structures, or spread to the blood as the fatal pyemia. Survival, while unlikely, occurred when the body was able to "wall off" the infection as an abscess. Also required for survival was a route for drainage of infected and inflammatory material to the outside, allowing the wound to slowly heal from the inside out. Sometimes such survival meant living with a chronic draining wound for the rest of the patient's life. The surgeon's role in these cases was most often a simple acceptance of his limitations.

Period Resource:

The Extraction of Bullets (and other foreign bodies)
from:
A Manual of Military Surgery— J. Julian Chisolm, M.D. (Evans and Cogwell, Columbia, 1864)

Notwithstanding all that has been written upon the innocuous character of balls embedded in the flesh, for every instance in which they have thus remained, without giving trouble, one hundred can be exhibited showing the great danger of foreign bodies in the living tissues. Baron Larrey's experience showed that, as a rule, amputations are eventually necessary, after years of suffering, in those cases in which balls have been left embedded in bones. These remarks are equally applicable to all foreign bodies, including spiculae of bone.
In McLeod's Surgery of the Crimea, the report of M. Hutin, chief surgeon of the Hotel des Invalides, is given, which is a striking commentary in favor of the removal of all foreign bodies. He reports that, of four thousand cases examined by him, in which balls had remained embedded, only twelve men suffered no inconvenience; and the wounds of two hundred continued to open and close until the foreign body was extracted.
The experience of the various hospital boards throughout the Confederacy for the examination of wounded soldiers on furlough, will attest the importance of M. Hutin's remarks. Very rarely is a soldier found returning to his regiment with a ball un-extracted, and in those cases in which the position of the foreign body escapes the careful examination of the surgical staff, painful and often contracted limbs are uniformly met with, rendering the patient totally unfit for service. When no doubt exists that a foreign body complicates the wound, the surgeon should neglect no precaution to discover it. As a general rule, he will find the examination facilitated by exposing the entire limb.
If the ball be felt loose in the soft parts, a bullet forceps can be made to seize it; and it can be extracted without difficulty, provided the disengaged hand of the surgeon support the limb on the opposite side

to that at which the forceps is introduced; otherwise, the ball glides in front of the forceps and can not be seized. The ordinary bullet forceps, simulating the dressing forceps of the pocked-case, was the instrument preferred by Larrey, and is still in general use. Many changes have been made in these, without advancing, to any extent, the merits of the instrument. An excellent bullet forceps, which is the one now issued in the Confederate service, terminates with a sharp prong on either blade, at right angles to the blade, so that, when closed, the points are protected by the blades. These act as an axis upon which the ball bay be rolled out of the wound, instead of being drawn out, as with the dressing forceps.

In my own experience, I have found an ordinary dissecting forceps, with toothed extremity, such as is met with in all recent pocket-cases, the most convenient instrument for extracting balls. The teeth, embedding themselves in the lead, allow of firm traction without fear of the instrument slipping, which is so constantly the case when the common bullet forceps is used. In removing a flattened ball, especially a mashed Miniè ball, a good deal of force is often required to disengage and extract the irregular mass from its bed in the soft parts. The long, ordinary bullet forceps is an unnecessarily clumsy instrument, made apparently with the belief that the ball will, in every instance, be sought for through a long tack of several inches, while rarely is this the case. The ball is usually found near the surface, and can be readily removed by a short-toothed forceps, which is much more conveniently handled.

Should the site of the foreign body be not at once evident after the examination of the wound, the limb should be carefully manipulated for some distance from the wound. As the object of the examination is to detect abnormal projections, the slightest elevation should attract attention. When no projection is visible, palpation may detect a hard body at a great depth in the tissues. The hand should, at first, be run lightly over the surface, as light pressure would expose the indurated spot, the site of a ball, when well defined pressure would move the object, push the ball back into its track, and cause its disappearance. If the tissues are soft, the foreign body can be seized between the fingers. If this be impossible, palpation over the region, as for detecting fluctuation, will discover the hard, resisting, circumscribed body. Experience soon makes perfect in this kind of research, and mistakes are rarely made.

Amputation

Amputation of an extremity (or part thereof) is necessary when the risk of the surgery is deemed less than the risk to life of treating the wound expectantly. In general, the risk of expectant treatment is higher when bone is shattered, when significant damage to a joint is caused by the wound, when extensive soft tissue damage renders the limb of little use, or when damage to major blood vessels causes hemorrhaging that cannot be controlled without depriving the limb of sufficient circulation for its survival.

The risk of the surgery is greater if it is delayed past 24 hours, by which time reaction has become fully established with swelling, heat, and discharge from the wound. The risk of the surgery is greater for amputation closer to the trunk (e.g. at the hip versus the thigh, and at the thigh versus the leg), and in general higher in the leg than in the arm. Also factoring into the decision is the transport that the patient must undergo, as a patient may be more easily and safely transported after an amputation than with a severe fracture or otherwise extensive extremity wound. Finally also to be considered, in a battlefield situation with thousands of wounded to be treated, is the time and nursing the wound will require if amputation is not resorted to. A wound that may be treated without amputation in civilian practice with a fair expectation of success may necessitate amputation on the battlefield.

The decision for amputation is based on this calculus for the simple and only purpose of preserving life.

Pictured below are the essential tools for a limb amputation. From above down, a large bone saw, a large single sided knife, a large double-sided knife (catlin), a bone file to smooth the cut bone end, and a tenaculum to capture and fix blood vessels to allow them to be ligated (tied off). Smaller tools were provided for use in the hand, foot, etc.

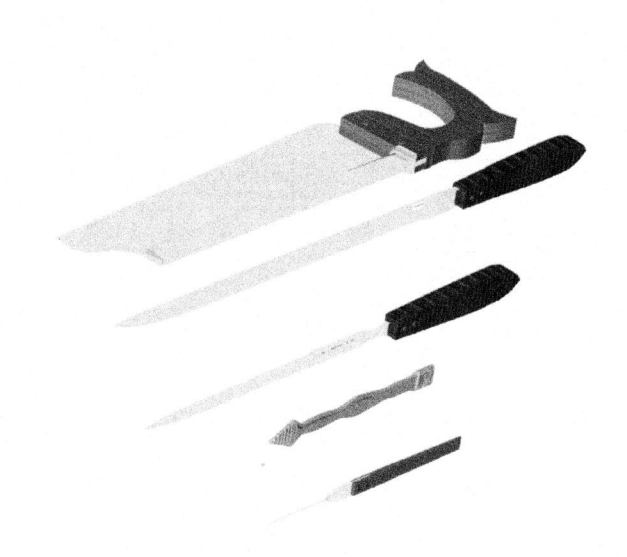

Bruce A. Evans, M.D.

Illustration (period text) of the circular method of amputation:

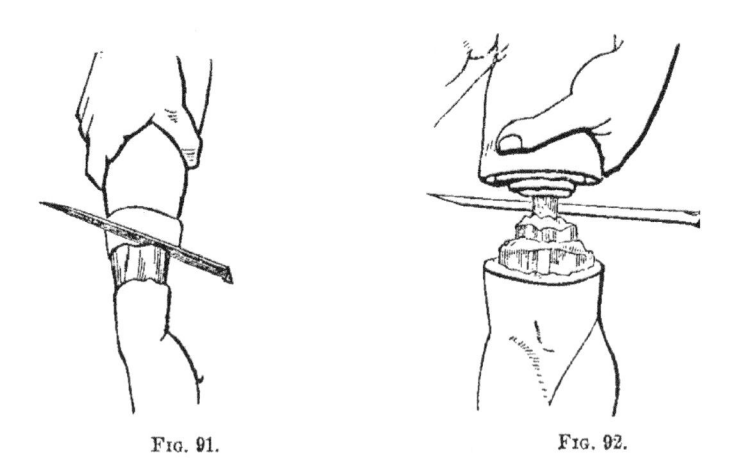

Fig. 91.

Fig. 92.

Illustration (period text) of the flap method of amputation:

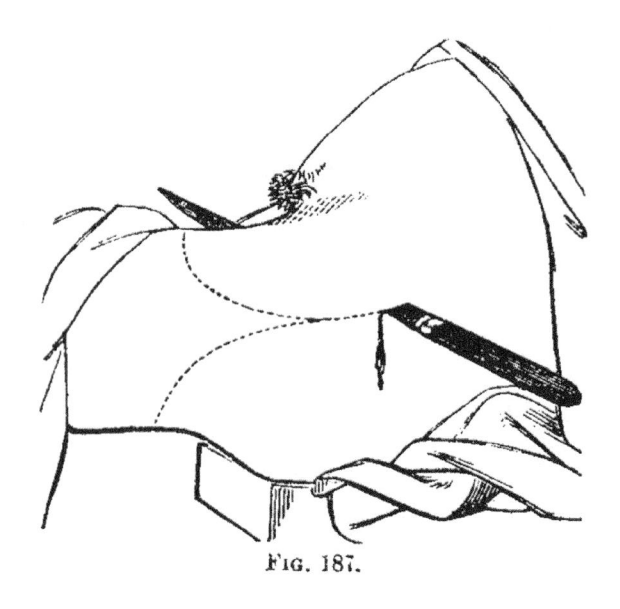

Fig. 187.

Modern Perspective:

Contemporary descriptions of piles of limbs outside of operating sites are numerous, symbolizing the horror of war. Almost 30,000 amputations were performed by Federal surgeons with a mortality rate of 26.3%. The frequency of amputations was due in part to the great frequency of extremity wounds. Another reason is that it was in the limbs, rather than the head and trunk, where the surgeon had at least an opportunity to improve upon the results of expectant treatment. This resulted directly from the lack on any method of dealing with what we now know are the effects of the universal presence of infection in the wound. Only in the extremity could this be dealt with by separation. The recognized indications for amputation correspond to those conditions in which life-threatening infection will almost invariably occur.

The major indication for amputation following extremity wounds was extensive bone or direct joint damage: the "shot fracture." The conoidal "ball" most commonly used had particular ability to fracture and splinter bone. Pulverized and splintered bone with many small fragments represented a major threat to survival without surgery. The wound would not heal unless the fragments of dead bone were removed, but extensive manipulation and exploration of the wound necessary to accomplish this, in the pre-antisepsis era, too often led to a poor result, with death from complications of "mortification", including pyemia, hospital gangrene, and secondary hemorrhage. Also, fractures involving a joint, or fractures associated with a great deal of soft tissue damage, would also prove fatal due to what are now known to be infectious complications if not treated with amputation. Finally, damage to a blood vessel necessary to the survival of the limb required amputation to avoid progressive death of tissue and the inevitable deadly mortification (dry gangrene).

The fatality rate for amputations in the lower leg was 33% and in the thigh 53%. In the thigh, the closer the amputation was to the hip, the higher the mortality. Amputations for hip fractures carried such a high mortality rate (more than 90%) that they were rarely performed, despite the untreated mortality of 83%.

Amputations were nearly exclusively performed with anesthesia, so operator speed was less important than in the pre-anesthetic days. This allowed time for careful technique. Anesthesia was light by modern standards, which allowed for remarkably few anesthesia deaths - given the simplicity of the technique and equipment - and rapid recovery of consciousness.

Overall, about one half of extremity shot fractures were treated with amputation. Two years after the end of the war, Lord Lister published an account of a compound fracture of the thigh - with exposure of the protruding bone to the atmosphere - treated by the use of carbolic acid dressings, setting the fracture, and allowing healing to take place. No mortification intruded. The era of antisepsis changed the arithmetic of amputation forever.

Period Resources:

Use of the Amputation Knife in Circular Amputation

from: Hand-Book of Surgical Operations — Steven Smith, M.D.(Bailliere, New York, 1862)

Circular Method.-There are three principal steps in this operation, viz. :1. Incision of the skin; 2. Incision of the muscles; 3. Section of the bone. To incise the skin easily and neatly, the operator should stand upon the right side of the limb, the left foot thrown forward and placed firmly upon the floor, the right knee bending sufficiently to give freedom of motion to the body; the left hand grasps the limb above the point of operation, and the handle of the knife is taken between the thumb and forefinger of the right hand, being lightly supported by the other fingers; stooping sufficiently to allow the right arm to encircle the limb readily, he carries the knife around until the blade is nearly perpendicular to the long axis of the limb on the side next to him with the point downwards, and the hand of the operator above the limb; he now commences the incision with the heel of the knife, giving slightly sawing motions, and brings the hand under the limb, and then directly upwards upon the side next to the operator, until the heel touches the point of commencement; the handle of the knife held thus delicately will change its relative positions as it passes around the limb without the slightest embarrassment to the operator; if the handle is firmly grasped in the whole hand, the incision cannot be completed without the aid of the other hand, or an awkward movement of the hand holding the knife; the ease with which the incision is completed will depend much upon whether it commences well down upon the side of the limb next to the operator. The skin is raised from the first layer of muscles by dissection, and drawn upwards, two or three inches, according to the diameter of the limb, like the cuff of a coat. 2. The first layer of muscles is divided at the margin of the retracted integument, in the same manner as the incision of the skin is executed; this layer is raised with the knife, and drawn still further upwards; and the last layer of muscles is divided down to the bone by the same sweep of the knife as before given.

Use of the Catlin Knife in Flap Amputations

from: Hand-Book of Surgical Operations — Steven Smith, M.D.(Bailliere, New York, 1862)

FLAPS.- Flaps may be anterior, posterior, or lateral; they may be made from without inwards, or from within outwards.
Single Flaps.-The operator grasps the tissues on the anterior part of the limb, with the left hand above the point of operation, and placing the heel of the knife (catlin) at the point of the fingers on the opposite side of the limb, with a slight downward curve, he brings it over to the point of the thumb on the opposite side, with one stroke dividing the tissues to the bone; he now withdraws the knife until the point rests in the angle of the wound, when he thrusts it under the bone, taking care

that the point emerges at the angle of the wound on the opposite side where the incision commenced; he now makes a flap from the posterior part of the limb of sufficient length to cover the stump; the muscles are dissected from the bone with the amputating knife or a scalpel; the operation is very rapid, the knife not being raised from the limb.

Double Flaps - The operator grasps the tissues on the upper part of the limb with the left hand, the thumb and fingers resting at the middle of the limb on opposite sides; the knife (catlin) is then entered at the thumb and thrust through above the bone, emerging on the opposite side at the point where the fingers rest, and passed downwards and outwards, c, making an anterior flap, b, of the required length; it is again re-entered at the same point, and passing beneath the bone emerges from the same point on the opposite side, and a flap is made from the posterior part of the limb; both flaps are forcibly retracted, the muscles dissected from the bone, and the bone divided.

Limb Conservation Surgery (Resection)

Limb conserving resection surgery is an alternative to amputation in some circumstances where expectant treatment cannot be undertaken. The technique usually involves the removal of an injured joint without removing the limb above the joint. Instead, a chain saw is used to cut the bones above and below the joint (if both joint surfaces are damaged) or below the joint with disarticulation of the now separated bone segment from the joint if only the lower surface was damaged.

If done carefully, and with excellent immobilization of the limb and nursing care through the long period of recovery, the results can be surprisingly good, with regrowth of bone in some circumstances giving a shortened and stiff but solid limb, and formation of a false joint with flexibility but little strength in others. Results are better in the upper extremity where weight bearing is not an issue and the importance of hand function may be preserved by the procedure.

The surgery is more difficult, takes longer, and requires more care in transport and nursing than amputation, all of which limit its use. It is most frequently used for shoulder and elbow injuries, especially by Confederate surgeons, who show more enthusiasm for its use than Federal surgeons, who have been generally disappointed with the results.

Bruce A. Evans, M.D.

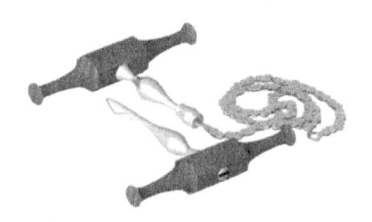

Pictured above is a chain saw used to resect damaged joints while preserving surrounding soft tissues

Pictured below is the placement of the chain saw for resection of a damaged joint, leaving the adjacent tissues intact and in continuity. The process would be performed above and below the joint to be removed. (period medical text)

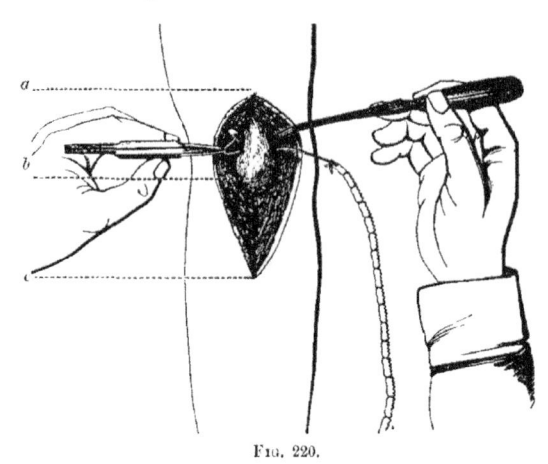

FIG. 220.

Modern Perspective:

An alternative to amputation that preserved some extremity function was resection. In this procedure, the injured part of the bone or an entire joint was cut away with a hand chain saw that could be passed around the bone without injuring other tissues. The resulting shortened limb was treated as a severe fracture, and could eventually reach a level of some useful function, if only to preserve a useful hand in an upper arm fracture, for instance. If performed skillfully, regrowth of bone connecting the resected ends was possible. There was a great deal of enthusiasm for resection in place of amputation in Confederate publications. The compiled experience of the Union surgeons was not supportive: in the upper extremity results were "disappointing" and in the lower extremity "disastrous", with mortality rates higher that for amputation, especially in the upper extremity. Resections of the shoulder and elbow were most resorted to. The high mortality for shoulder amputation made resection an attractive option, especially in the view of Confederate surgeons. Unfortunately, resection required more skilled operators, a longer operating time, and long periods of immobilization of the limb not possible with primitive transportation. All these factors likely were responsible for the fact that only 14% of extremity shot fractures treated surgically were treated with limb-conserving resection.

It was not through indifference that such decisions were made, although a conservative tendency on the part of surgeons, especially in the Federal service, likely did play a role.

Period Resource:

Limb Conservation with Joint Resection in Place of Amputation from:
A Manual of Military Surgery— J. Julian Chisolm, M.D. (Evans and Cogwell, Columbia, 1864)
For injury to the heads of bones forming the joints in the upper extremity resection is particularly applicable, and this operation is now the rule of practice, having superseded amputation in all cases where the blood-vessels and nerves around the joint are not involved in the

injury. When a joint has in any way been injured by a gunshot wound, whether the joint has been largely opened, or the heads of the bones forming the articulation crushed, as soon as the excessive shock under which the patient may be suffering passes off, we proceed at once to operate. A primary resection is as much called for as a primary amputation, and is followed by as successful results. It should be performed within twenty-four or thirty-six hours, 0r before reaction sets in. Such eases would do much better if the patient could be transferred to the general hospital prior to an operation, as transportation is difficult and dangerous immediately after the resection, from the difficulty of securing the limb from movements. Experience has so established this fact that, in cases necessitating a long and tedious transportation, the rule is to amputate rather than to resect, inasmuch as the gravity of the resection is very much increased by the transportation. Should the case not come under observation until reaction has set in, then, by general, mild, antiphlogistic treatment, and ice bladders or cold water dressings locally, we await the establishment of suppuration-after which the operation might be attempted with good prospects of success.

The results of the primary resection are more successful than the secondary; and these are, in turn, much more likely to succeed than when the operation is performed during the stage of febrile excitement. There are three or four rules necessary in all cases of resection, and which should not be forgotten during the operation, viz: Make the incisions for exposing the heads of the bones in that portion of the extremity opposite to the main blood-vessels and nerves, so that these may not be exposed to injury. If possible, make the existing wound lie in the line of operations, and place the incisions in such a way as to permit a continued drain from the joint. Make these incisions free, so as not to cramp the operator in turning out the heads of the bones. An inch added to the incision does not increase its serious character, and hastens the operation. Remove most of the synovial membrane, and save as much periosteum as possible; the one is prone to take on inflammation - the other makes, and will, to a certain extent, reproduce the bone. In performing secondary resections, the removal of all the diseased synovial membrane becomes one of the first elements for success.

More successes are obtained from resections of the shoulder-joint than from an operation upon any other articulation - the statistical tables of the final results of operations in favor of resection being conclusive over amputations [at that joint].

In examining [the data] take into consideration that primary operations are performed upon the most serious injuries; the cases of apparently trivial injury are kept, and resection found necessary during the progress of the case.

When the ball has entered directly within a joint, only the surface may require excision; but should the head of the bone be extensively spiculated, we must cut back to the sound bone, even if we are compelled to remove four or five inches of the shaft of a bone, as was successfully done first by Stromyer for a gunshot injury, and several times in the Confederate service. Should the receiving cavity be equally injured, the fractured portion should be removed. The rule is, never to remove more of the bone than is absolutely called for, and not to open the medullary [marrow] cavity if it can in any way be avoided. When the wound has been cleansed of all foreign bodies, the flap is replaced and secured with one or two points of suture. As adhesion by the first intention is not usually expected, and gives no advantage over the final result by granulation, nice adjustment along the entire line of the incision is not necessary. An opening must be left at the most dependent portion of the wound for drainage. The patient is then put to bed, and cold water dressings applied. Inflammation at first runs high, the parts around the joint are much swollen, and a collection soon forms within the cavity from which the bones have been removed. The escape of this decomposed blood and pus from the wound gives great relief. When kept in by the too nice adjustment of the flap, the collection increases the swelling, oedema, and pain, which is diffused over the neighboring parts, involving the chest as well as arm. When suppuration becomes established the swelling and pain subside, granulations spring up, and eventually close the wound. In the meantime, the divided muscles have formed new relations. By means of the lymphy exudation they become more or less incorporated with the surrounding tissues, and, by attaching themselves around the cut portion of the bone form, in time, a closed capsule. A head to the bone is sometimes, in a measure, formed; in other cases the end of the bone becomes attached to the cavity by fibrinous bands.

As suppuration will be excessive and often long continued, nourishment and stimuli will be required during the treatment, When abscesses form in the surrounding cellular tissue they should be opened. It is a matter of but little importance in what position the limb is placed, and how it is secured, provided its position is comfortable to the sufferer. The uneasiness and irritation which the splints and bandages give, do much to prevent success. In the upper extremity it matters little what length of limb the patient has, provided his life be saved and the convalescence be speedy. A shortened arm does not affect its usefulness, and a slightly changed direction can be corrected in the after-stages of the treatment. The most effectual management is the simplest and tedious daily dressings are to be discouraged. Straightening the limb upon the bed, a pillow, or a long, broad splint, without complicated or elaborate bandaging, is the best and most comfortable dressing for any resection. The patient is kept in bed until the suppurative stage is established, when he will be permitted to get up. His arm is then placed in a sling, and the water dressings are continued until a complete cure is effected. When the parts are nearly cicatrized it will be time enough to apply the tumefaction bandage for removing the oedema of the limb. Anchylosis rarely follows this operation in the shoulder joint.

Of the eases of resection of the shoulder performed in the Crimea but few died; and all those saved regained a useful limb, possessing all the motions, with the exception of those of the deltoid, which muscle is, to a certain extent, paralyzed from the division of its nerves, which can not altogether be avoided in exposing the head of the bone. As a proof of the efficacy of resection, Stromyer excised nineteen shoulder-joints with a loss of seven, chiefly from pyemia. Of eight cases in which the operation was required, but, from some mitigating circumstances, was not performed, five died.

Head Wounds

Penetrating wounds of the head, involving damage to the brain, are frequently fatal. Experience has adequately shown that the chances of survival are not improved by surgical treatment beyond the examination necessary to establish the facts. Whether the wound involves soft tissue only, or involves penetration of the skull and the brain and its covering membranes, operative procedures are therefore not undertaken by experienced surgeons beyond the usual examination and removal of foreign objects from the soft tissue wounds.

Wounds resulting in skull fractures in which pieces of broken bone press on the brain causing symptoms of paralysis or coma are sometimes treated by removal of a disk of bone through trephination allowing the introduction of an instrument to lift or elevate the bone piece relieving the pressure. Although improvement sometimes occurs, too often the result, after an encouraging delay, is the onset of cerebral fever and death. Many argue, therefore, against the use of trephination.

Wounds of the head directly penetrating the brain through the tough fibrous covering of the dura mater are almost invariably fatal. A soldier with such a wound who survives long enough to arrive at the field hospital succumbs within hours, or a day or two at the most. The pitiful victims of such wounds, consequently, are usually kept comfortable as the inevitable end approaches. From a sense of powerlessness and frustration, a surgeon may not keep himself from attempting to intervene.

Modern Perspective:

Bruce A. Evans, M.D.

With a few exceptions fractures of the skull caused by wounds were treated conservatively. Surgery was attempted only if a piece of bone from the inner table of the skull was felt to be pressing into the brain, or if a fracture lay over the course of a major skull artery in a patient showing signs of deterioration from bleeding on the brain.

The poor results of either exploration or trephination under battlefield conditions led most to a conservative approach. In trephination, a disk of skull is removed by a circular saw apparatus to allow access to the space between the skull and the dura mater, a tough lining around the brain. With that access, depressed fractures could be elevated, splintered fragments of bone removed, bleeding arteries underlying the skull ligated, and rarely hemorrhage between the skull and the dura drained. The results however, were poor, with 45% of the patients dying. This was often worse than expectant treatment.

With regard to penetrating injuries of the brain, immediate death resulted from damage to portions of the brain controlling vital bodily functions, or from massive bleeding causing secondary pressure on those structures. Delayed death resulted either from swelling of the brain tissue associated with the injury causing similar pressure, or from infection caused by the presence of foreign bodies in the brain tissue. Effective treatment was beyond the knowledge of the time. Any treatment, including probing for and removal of the missile and any foreign matter propelled into the wound by its violent entrance, were futile, as additional deterioration from swelling and further cause of infection only hastened the end.

Period Resource:

Surgery for Penetrating Head Wounds and Skull Fracture
from:
A Manual of Military Surgery— J. Julian Chisolm, M.D. (Evans and Cogwell, Columbia, 1864

[The types of head wounds are:]
1. Injury to the soft parts alone, uncomplicated with injury to skull or brain.
2. Wound of soft parts, with simple fracture of the skull.
3. Wound with depressed fracure of the skull, but without symptoms of compression.
4. Compound depresssed fracture of the skull, with symptoms of compression of the brain.
5. Perforating wounds of the skull, complicated with foreign bodies in the brain.

[The first 3 and the 5th are never treated with operation. Experience has shown that, in the case of the first 3 it is unneccessary and recovery most often ensues, and in the last it only hurries the usual fatal issue.]

The fourth variety of injury to the head, and by far the most serious [of the first four], is that in which a compound fracture, with depressed fragments, is connected with symptoms of compression and paralysis. This is the only variety of complicated head wounds in which surgeons now consider instrumental interference justifiable; and even in this instance, although no doubt exists that, in some cases immediate relief has followed the lifting of the depressed bone, the propriety of trephining, as rule, is doubted by many army surgeons of large experience. The successful treatment of such injuries will depend more upon the condition of the brain and membranes than merely upon the depression. Should these be lacerated, or in any way injured, inflammation will probably show itself, sooner or later, The operation of trephining, under such circumstances, would increase the local irritation, expose the injured tissues to injurious atmospheric influences, and hasten on a violent, and usually fatal, inflammation.
If the brain and membranes be not injured, experience teaches that the brain will soon become accustomed to the pressure; and, although insensibility may continue for hours, days, or, as in many instances of ultimate recovery, for weeks, the symptoms of compression and paralysis will gradually pass off. By not using instruments, the surgeon

has the satisfaction of knowing that he has not increased the local trouble by a serious operation. When the depressed bone is not raised, the removal of the symptoms of compression, being very gradual, excessive reaction is not likely to follow; and as no air has been admitted to the effusions beneath the skull, the probability of suppuration will be much diminished. When effusions have taken place, the depressed bone acts as a covering, excluding air, with its injurious chemical influences; and autopsies at some distant period show that fluids, uncontaminated by decomposition, can be absorbed. When the skull is opened, and the free admission of air is permitted, suppuration, with, perhaps, pyemia, is prone to occur.

Stromyer, who is one of the highest authorities on gunshot wounds of the head, and who, as surgeon-in-chief of the Schleswig-Holstein army, had every facility for studying his favorite branch of surgery, gives us, as the result of his experience, observation, and study, that the trephine can be abandoned in military surgery. In a supplement to his work on Military Surgery, recently published, he states: " That in military surgery trephining is never needed. When the case is so severe as to require the trephine in gunshot wounds, the patient will die in spite of it." In the last two campaigns, in which he had charge of the army, he has not trephined. Loeffler, a distinguished surgeon in the Prussian service, who has published one of the best books of instruction for military surgeons, after acknowledging Stromyer as the master in all relating to the treatment of gunshot wounds of the head, endorses his views in opposition to trephining.

McLeod gives the following as the Crimean experience: "As to the use of the trephine - the cases and time for its application - less difference of opinion, I believe, exists among the experienced army surgeons than among civilians; and I think the decided tendency among them is to endorse the modern treatment by expectancy, and to avoid operating except in rare cases. In this, I believe, they judge wisely; for when we examine the question carefully, we find that there is not one single indication for having recourse to operations which cannot, by the adduction of pertinent cases, be shown to be often fallacious." Hewett, in a series of lectures on injuries of the head, published in the Medical Times and Gazette for 1859, which form the most complete treatise extant on the subject, is equally adverse to the trephine. Guthrie, Cole, and Williamson, in their reports, equally confirm the dangers of the trephine, and the great fatality accompanying its use.

The entire records of the science may be searched in vain to find a duplicate series of successful cases to that reported by Steornyer. Of forty-one cases of fracture, with depression from gunshot wounds, in many of which it was probable that the brain and membranes were injured, only seven died-all the rest recovered. In only one case was there any operative interference, although signs of secondary compression appeared in several. The antiphlogistic treatment, carefully carried out, was alone adhered to.

No surgeon can doubt that the operation of trephining has cost many a man his life; and although many
cases have recovered after the operation, it is a question whether, in the majority of cases, more rapid recovery would not have been obtained without it.

When symptoms of compression, accompanied with paralysis, and, finally, finally, stupor, ensue in the course of treatment, continue the steady, onward use of antiphlogistic remedies. At this juncture many surgeons recommend calomel pushed to salivation, which some state to be synonymous with salvation. There is, however, no unanimity on this head; the modern practice is to treat such cases without the use of mercury.

At this stage of the case, which is one of extreme gravity, a successful course of treatment can hardly be expected. Should the symptoms of compression have been preceded by one or more severe chills, with excitement of the pulse, pain in the head, divergence of the eyes, protrusion of the tongue to one side, a dull, pricking sensation in the arm and leg opposite to that wounded, we might feel assured that pus, or some effused fluid, has been thrown out upon the brain, and, usually, that the substance of this organ has become more or less softened. As such cases are exceedingly fatal, the operation of trephining is usually performed, hoping that the collection of pus may be found and discharged, and that, by the relief of pressure, the serious symptoms may be also removed. Very rare instances of such successes are upon record, but in by far the majority of cases the symptoms continue unabated, even when the abscess has been opened.

Penetrating Chest Wounds

Penetrating chest wounds, while not invariably fatal, do not seem to benefit from any particular treatment - other than the usual wound examination and care - or surgical intervention. The mortality is highest when it is clear that the lung itself has been directly damaged. This is indicated by signs such as shortness of breath, bubbling of air from the wound, and coughing up blood. Some of these patients survive, usually with slowly healing wounds draining infected matter. Many die - probably more than 70%. Spurred by the bubbling of air through the wounds and the obvious breathing difficulty of many patients, some surgeons advocate sealing the wounds with airtight materials such as rubberized dressings and collodium soaked patches. Although this often benefits the respiratory distress, careful following of the patients so treated indicates that unless the dressing is removed they are more likely to die in the end, many with pyemia.

Modern Perspective:

Many chest wounds led to quick death on the battlefield. Death from rapid blood loss or loss of heart function was attendant on direct heart damage or damage to the aorta carrying blood from the heart, or other large arteries. Pentrating wounds of both lungs leading to collapse of both lungs caused rapid suffication and death.

Penetrating wounds of the lung cavity, with or without direct lung damage, endanger life initially though collapse and respiratory failure, and later through infections of the sterile space around the lungs or of the lung tissue itself - pneumonia. If enough respiratory function remained to keep the patient alive, and a pathway remained for drainage of pus from the inevitable infection, survival was possible but unlikely (70% died). Although the patch technique sometimes relieved some of the respiratory distress of the lung-shot soldier by preventing air leakage, without an external drainage pathway for infected matter, internal infection eventually took the patient's life, occasionally after a prolonged and enervating struggle.

Penetrating Abdominal Wounds

Penetrating wounds of the abdomen are frequently fatal. Experienced surgeons know that the chances of survival are not improved by surgical treatment beyond the usual examination of the wound.

Therefore, a surgeon is in a position of impotence when faced with soldiers with penetrating bullet wounds of the abdomen. Unlike with brain wounds however, these patients are conscious to near the end, with considerable suffering. Free use of morphine or opium is indicated. These wounds are also accompanied by an almost insatiable thirst. Unfortunately, with a stomach or bowel wound drinking water seems to increase the ultimate suffering. The speed at which the end is reached depended mainly on the extent of bowel injury and the consequent fecal soiling of the abdomen.

Modern Perspective:

Infection of the abdomen or peritonitis is almost inevitable in penetrating abdominal wounds and almost invariably fatal if no intervention is undertaken. Once again, however, without antisepsis and antibiotics any effort of the contemporary surgeon only made things worse. J.E.B. Stuart died "in his own blood and feces" in a bed in Richmond 27 hours after his wound received at Yellow Tavern. With his abdomen pierced below the ribs on the left side, he was able to reminisce and resign himself to God's will. The inevitable end was known to all from the start.

On the other hand, some apparently fatal wounds such as the pelvic wound received by J.L.Chamberlain at Petersburg the same year, were occasionally survived, sometimes through a daring and creative surgical effort. Following his battlefield elevation to brevet Brigadier General occasioned by his expected death, friends of Chamberlain objected to the decision to simply await his death. Two regimental surgeons, Shaw and Townsend, reconstructed his torn urethra and reattached it to his damaged bladder, working around a silver catheter inserted through the urethra into the bladder. His life was saved, although the rest of his long life was plagued by leaking urine and recurrent infections.

Soft Tissue Wounds

Most soft tissue wounds involve the arms and legs, since they represent the major exposure of the body to enemy fire. Soft tissue wounds of the extremities sparing the bones and joints rarely carry a risk of death and when involving the extremities rarely lead to a consideration of amputation. Exceptions include extensive soft tissue damage rendering the limb more burden than asset, or damage to major arteries of an extent preventing an adequate blood supply to the limb. Over 50,000 soft tissue injuries to the lower extremity have been reported to the Union Medical Department during this war. Only 201 of these resulted in amputation, and many of these were secondary procedures performed after the development of hospital gangrene or traumatic erysipelas in the limb. The other main cause is destruction of major arteries by the original injury.

For most of these wounds, once they have been examined and probed and any foreign bodies removed, expectant treatment is the rule. The mortality of flesh wounds varies by area, ranging from 14% in the neck to 1% in the chest.

Modern Perspective:

Wounds of the soft tissues, without involvement of sterile body cavities, bones, or joints, were the most survivable of wounds.
An adequate examination and removal of the bullet and any clothing or other foreign objects driven into the wound were necessary to promote healing.
These wounds all, from a modern perspective, were infected. Without antibiotics, the patient's natural defenses were all that existed to fight off the infection. Generally, for that reason, the

wounds healed best "by second intention", that is by gradually filling in from the bottom with healing "granulation tissue", which allowed drainage of pus produced by the infection from the wound until the wound gradually healed. If an attempt was made to heal the wound "by first intention" - by bringing the lips of the exterior wound together, trimming the edges for a good fit if necessary, the danger of a deep infection, unable to drain, becoming a chronic abscess was increased. This could lead to pyemia (blood poisoning) and death. If an abscess continued to drain pus through the skin through a pathway - called a sinus or fistula - this was best treated by opening in up using a director and a knife, and allowing healing from the inside out with enhanced opportunities for drainage.

Probing Bullet Wounds

The best probe is the finger - it is less likely to damage tissue than metal probes and the sense of touch not transmitted by such probes is crucial. To identify the bullet track and find retained missiles, it is sometimes necessary to arrange the limbs in their position at the time of the injury.

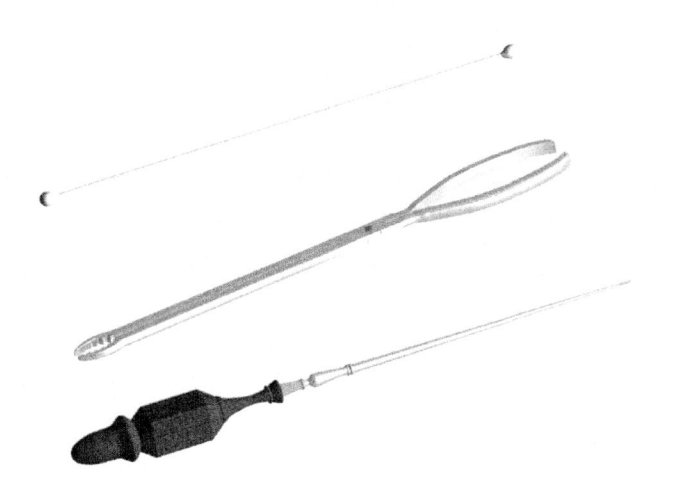

Pictured here are (from above) a Nealton bullet probe (having ceramic ends meant to be marked by the lead of a bullet to verify it was not touching bone alone), a forceps-type bullet extractor, and an extractor with a threaded end meant to screw into a bullet and allow its removal (not a successful instrument in most surgeons' hands).

Modern Perspective:

Unfortunately, the lack of knowledge of the causes of wound infection and the resultant lack of knowledge of antiseptic or aseptic surgical practices, meant that any probing of the wound was likely to contaminate it.

Nevertheless, given that under the circumstances every wound would be infected, it was true (and remains so even in the antibiotic era) that foreign bodies retained in the wound would likely cause persistent infection and result in non-healing, chronically draining wounds at best, or death from blood poisoning at worst. Therefore, the practice of carefully probing the wounds for foreign bodies (bullets, bits of clothing pushed into the wound ahead of the bullets) as well as shattered bits of bone (which, once dead, act in the same fashion as a foreign body) and removing them if found was appropriate surgical practice.

Given that nothing was clean in an antiseptic sense, the common practice of using a finger for a probe where possible due to the sensory feedback, which draws appalled attention from current historians, probably resulted in less damage to the wounds and better determination of the presence and location of foreign bodies than metal probes.

When necessary, these examinations were carried out under anesthesia.

Period Resource:

The Use of Probes in Gunshot Wounds
from: A Manual of Military Surgery— J. Julian Chisolm, M.D. (Evans and Cogwell, Columbia, 1864)

As soon as the wounded arrive at the temporary resting-place or field infirmary, where the surgeons are assembled, all bandages are removed, and the wounds carefully examined. A glance at the wound, when the clothing has been previously inspected, will often tell, when there are two orifices differing in appearance and in a direct line with each other, whether foreign bodies have lodged or not. As the patient is now faint from loss of blood and from nervous depression, the wound not yet being painful or swollen, the surgeon, using his index finger - which is the only admissible probe on such occasions that the military surgeon of experience recognizes - examines with it, if possible, the entire extent of the wound, searching for foreign bodies. Where the orifice is too small to admit the index finger, the little finger will be found equally serviceable, and by flattening the limb, by making pressure upon the side opposite to and against the finger, a much greater extent of the wound can be explored.

This examination is made without fear of reproducing hemorrhage, as the finger can not displace the clots which hold firmly to the openings in the vessel. Every surgeon has noticed how rudely a stump might be sponged, and what force it requires to wipe away clots which have formed over the face of a smooth, incised, open wound. The adhesions are increased a hundred-fold by the irregularities of a concealed bullet track. The finger finds no difficulty in entering a hole through which a bullet has passed, if examined, as every wound ought to be, before swelling has taken place.

In examining fresh wounds, a silver probe will travel in the direction given to it by the surgeon; and as most persons guide the probe instead of allowing the probe to guide them, the true course of a ball can only be determined by it with great difficulty. It is but recently that I saw a physician of experience, in seeking the course of a ball which had lodged in the thigh, pass the probe, apparently without effort, among the muscles quite across the limb, so that, the bullet wound being on the outer side of the thigh, the end of the probe could be felt under the skin on its inner side. When the finger was introduced, it followed the track of the ball at a very oblique course from the one which the probe had taken. This example, which is only one of the many of frequent occurrence, is sufficient to show why military surgeons of experience denounce the silver probe, and distinguish by its use the tyro in surgical practice.

In those cases only in which, from the small size of the orifice made by pistol balls, the finger can not be introduced, is a large bulbed ball probe, a female catheter, or, lastly, an ordinary silver probe, used. Elastic bougies have been recommended for the examination of extensive wounds, but they are apt to bend should they meet an obstacle or irregularity in the track and when used for detecting foreign bodies do not convey the same satisfactory information as do metallic instruments.

The wound is examined from both sides, with the double object of finding foreign bodies which may have lodged, and seeing the proximity of the course of the ball to the main arteries of the limb. It is a matter of importance to determine the condition of large vessels, whether they be injured or not, by examining the degree of pulsation which they possess, as such an injury would necessitate a more careful after-treatment, in order to prevent secondary hemorrhage.

In some cases the finger introduced into the opening, after passing through the skin and cellular tissue, finds no further passage. This sudden arrest of the finger would indicate either that the ball had been drawn out with the removal of the clothing, or that the deep tissues, muscles, and aponeuroses have changed their relations on account of changes in the position of the limb. The track of the ball will not be discovered until the former relations of the parts be resumed, by placing the limb in the same position in which it had received the injury, when the entire route of the ball will be traced.

The inexperienced, readily deceived by the little resistance met with in probing recent wounds, mistaking muscular interstices for the track of the ball, make several false passages in their search for the foreign body, and by their isolation or denudation of the parts cause inflammation and add to the difficulties of further examination. When the finger, buried in the wound, shows that it is continued beyond reach, a ball probe or silver catheter, introduced carefully and without force, will often reach and detect the foreign body.

In the examination of gunshot wounds, to detect the presence of a ball, when, by the use of a silver ball probe, a hard foreign body is discovered, but from the depth of the wound and the little play of the bulb of the probe, it is impossible to determine whether we are feeling an exposed portion of bone or cartilage, or have actually found the foreign body which we are seeking, we can at once solve our doubts and establish an accurate diagnosis by means of Nealton's probe, which differs from the ordinary ball probe in having an unglazed porcelain bulb at its extremity. When this bulb, buried in the depth of a gunshot wound, reaches the suspected foreign body, it is only necessary to rotate it a few times against the hard mass and then withdraw it; when, if it has been rubbed against a lead ball, its surface will be blacked by particles of the metal, which discoloration can be produced by no other substance. This simple instrument is a triumph of surgical ingenuity.

Shot Fractures

When fractures are present, a judgement must be made whether the type of fracture and the extent of bone and tissue damage necessitates amputation for an increased chance at survival. Limb conservation surgery - resection - that might be possible in a civilian practice may be excluded, especially in the lower extremity, based on lack of time when faced with great numbers, gentle transport, and nursing care. If the limb may be saved, treatment is as for soft tissue wounds except that a careful attempt must be made to remove free pieces of bone, or chronic discharge of pus instead of healing will result.

Penetrating wounds of the head, chest, and abdomen are rarely benefited by operative treatment, and those who may survive do so with expectant and supportive care.

Modern Perspective:

When a wound involves injury to bone the mortality rate immediately increases compared to an injury of the soft tissues alone. Fractures associated with penetrating gunshot wounds are by definition compound fractures, defined as a fracture exposed to the air through a skin defect. Any compound fracture is a serious danger to life. If the bone is actually protruding from the skin and freely exposed to the atmosphere, the danger is extreme and amputation often indicated to save life.

The examination of the wound is crucial both to the decision as to whether amputation is necessary to increase the chance of survival and to remove foreign bodies, including pieces of separated bone, to allow healing to occur if the decision for a conservative treatment course is made. Extensive crushing of the bone into many small fragments or more than incidental involvement of the joint capsule argues strongly for amputation (or, in some circumstances, limb conservation resection) to increase the likelihood of survival.

If the fracture is simple, once foreign objects are removed, the wound may be treated in the usual fashion. The patient will require splinting, both to encourage healing into a strong bone and to minimize, to the extent possible, the severe pain that accompanies travel in wagons of patients with fractures. Simple battlefield splints with pieces of wood bound with bandages to the limb are rarely effective; in a general hospital more effective and elaborate machinery such as Smith's anterior splint may be utilized.

Erysipelas

Erysipelas can occur spontaneously – often involving the face – or complicate any wound. It occurs in 0.4 per thousand shot wounds.

Inflammation of the skin is associated with scarlet hue and firm swelling, originating from a wound, and quickly extending over the surrounding parts associated with a high fever, and ending in rapid loss of tissue. The spread is primarily local, but suppuration (pus formation) in the axillary or inguinal lymph glands can occur. The disease onset is associated with severe prostration. The average duration is 11 days. Multiple attacks are possible, with subsequent attacks likely to be more virulent. The mortality is high at 41%, including the mortality due to wound itself and other complications. The spread of this complication is clearly contagious. Isolation of the patient is called for as soon as the disease is identified. A ward with good ventilation is required. Destruction of all contaminate articles including clothing is undertaken. Precautions are required as for gangrene, including no use of sponges and dressings transferred from one patient to another.

Medical treatment is similar in spontaneous or wound-related erysipelas. The primary treatment is prevention through isolation of cases, non-reuse of dressings, &c. Tincture of Iodine (prepared with alcohol from Pannier #4) is applied to the wound, and cloths soaked with creosote (Pannier #46) to surrounding parts. Internal treatment includes quinine for fever (Pannier #34) and muriate of iron (Pnnier#50), felt by some to be almost a specific treatment. A supportive diet is used, rather than a low, depletion diet used in many inflammatory diseases, due to the universally expected transition to prostration.

The Practice of Civil War Medicine and Surgery

Modern Perspective:

This is a superficial skin infection caused by Streptococcus, which is often self-limited but if untreated can be fatal. As was recognized, it may occur spontaneously, in which case the infection usually involves the face and head. It may also complicate any wound. The advocated treatments were likely not effective, and the universal enthusiasm for muriate of iron as a specific treatment is somewhat mystifying.

It is highly contagious, and the same preventative procedures found to be effective in preventing the spread of hospital gangrene were found to be effective in this case. A significant advance regarding germ theory and antiseptic use of "disinfectants" could have been suggested by this knowledge.

Period Reference:

Erysipelas — Compiled from Various Medical Sources

Erysipelas may complicate any wound, or may occur spontaneously.
Spontaneous Erysipelas
The onset is usually with chills and fever except in mild cases. Within a few hours there appears the erysipelous blush, usually involving the nose, cheek, or ear. This is followed by a rapid spreading of the blush with swelling (enough to close eyes), increased fever, occasionally delirium, and finally bullae formation (blistering). Within a few to 6-7 days, scabbing, desquamation (peeling off of skin), decreased swelling and decreased fever develop. Occasionally, recovery is delayed due to dysentery. Initially a sthenic disease, but if it becomes prolonged it clearly has an adynamic character. If fatal, the symptoms are accompanied by the rapid development of coma and petechiae (skin bleeding). Complications of erysipelas include a discharge from the ears leading to deafness, parotid abscess in the neck, pneumonia, and potentially fatal cerebral inflammation (especially spread from orbits

or diffuse scalp involvement).

The disease is increased in winter. It has been clearly recognized as contagious as it was noted that adjacent patients would contract the disease, as would the nurses caring for them. This has led to use of isolation wards.

Treatment

Isolation of the patient is called for as soon as the disease is identified. A ward with good ventilation is required. Destruction of all contaminated articles including clothing is undertaken. When sthenic features predominate (increased excitement of system) treatment includes salines, laxatives, diaphoretics, and purgatives (especially if cerebral symptoms are present). Tincture of iron felt to be almost a specific treatment, taken internally. If the pulse weak, or low, muttering delirium is present (that is, asthenic features predominate) treatment should include a stimulating diet (beef essence, milk, especially alcohol). Local treatment includes oil, lard, or glycerin to exclude air from the lesions for comfort, tincture of iodine painted on, or silver nitrate, tincture of iron or persulphate of iron solution. Lancing or draining of the abscesses sometimes performed.

Hemorrhage

Life itself often depends upon the surgeon's action is controlling hemorrhage.

Pressure is one of the most constant resources of surgery for control of bleeding.

It may be done with the fingers, relieving one hand when fatigued by supporting it with the other. The point chosen is one where the artery involved may be pressed against bone.

The *tourniquet,* as used in amputations, or in any operations endangering the vessels, may be employed to arrest haemorrhage. The strap of webbing, with a buckle and pad, constitutes what is called the *field tourniquet,* several of which are supplied in every army surgeon's case of instruments. A *ligature* may be applied either to the wounded portion of the artery, or at a point nearer the heart, the vessel being laid bare by an incision made for the purpose. In order to secure the end of an artery in a wound, a hook or tenaculum may be inserted in it, or it may be grasped with a pair of forceps. We may generally look for the separation of ligatures from the fifth to the twelfth day after that of their application; it is due to the destructive ulceration of the vessel at the strictured point. *Styptic medications,* causing not only coagulation of the flowing blood, but contraction of the wounded tissues and their vessels, are very often indispensable. Thus, in cases of wounds in the cavity of the upper maxillary bone, in the rectum, fauces, etc., we often cannot depend upon any other means. Styptics may be used either in the solid form or in solution; they are perhaps most efficient when powdered. Much in vogue as a styptic is the persulphate of iron, commonly called Monsel's salt; it may be used either in substance or in strong solution, and not only causes immediate coagulation of the blood, but is in a great measure free from the caustic property so objectionable in other remedies of the kind.

See the next section on secondary hemorrhage for *Modern Perspective* and Period Resources on treatment of hemorrhage.

Secondary Hemorrhage

Secondary hemorrhage is a feared complication of wounds or amputations. It represents uncontrolled arterial hemorrhage at a time remote from the initial injury, which may or may not have involved ligation for primary hemorrhage control. Secondary hemorrhage complicating the recovery from amputation may occur spontaneously, or occur at the time of attempted removal of the ligatures from the stump.

Treatment is by ligation of an artery above (closer to the heart) the site of the bleeding, after initial control with pressure if possible. Mortification of a limb or stump (dry gangrene) may supervene if such ligation deprives the limb of sufficient blood to sustain vitality.

Amputation (at a higher level if amputation has already been performed) is the treatment of last resort. The mortality of these emergent procedures in the presence of severe hemorrhage is high.

Modern Perspective:

Wounds directly damaging arteries threatened life through primary hemorrhage. Control of the bleeding by tourniquet or pressure might allow a soldier to reach the field hospital, but more permanent treatment would be required for survival. The usual treatment was an operative approach to tie off (ligate) the artery in the wound, or above the wound. Some wounds were fatal because of damage to an artery that could not be ligated, either because of a deep or otherwise inaccessible location, or because the blood supply of the artery was necessary for other vital structures. Some patients died because of shock (circulatory collapse) due to cumulative loss of blood volume despite eventual control of hemorrhage. Many died with recurrent hemorrhage, either immediately due to inadequate control of the damaged artery, or later—secondary hemorrhage —as the ligated artery sloughed away during the "healing" process due, in most cases, to weakening of the wall of the artery or a clot by persistent infection. Although victims were treated with various stimulants and tonics, there was no way to increase the blood volume directly, and patients died who in later years would have been saved with blood transfusions or intravenous fluids. Interestingly, it had been known in India that patients dying of cholera (who essentially die of shock due to fluid loss from the bowels) could be almost miraculously revived from the edge of death by introduction of salt fluids into the vein. However, they would then die within 24 hours of blood poisoning (pyemia). This fate is, to us, unsurprising given the non-sterile nature of the fluids introduced. Direct treatment of shock therefore remained out of reach.

Period Resource:

The Control of Hemorrhage and Use of Tourniquets for Gunshot Wounds

from: A Manual of Military Surgery— J. Julian Chisolm, M.D. (Evans and Cogwell, Columbia, 1864)

If the hemorrhage be free, immediately after the receipt of injury, the best mode of controlling it would be the application of a ball of lint, a compress, or sponge over the wound, secured by a bandage, which, in closing the outer orifice, favors the formation of a clot. If the hemorrhage is at all active, as from some large artery, in addition to the compress on the wound, the entire limb should be carefully enveloped in a bandage, to some distance above the injury, so that the pressure made upon the soft parts would diminish the amount of circulating fluid in the limb, and prevent the ingress of blood into the tissues. The haemostatic properties of this dressing are very much increased by soaking the sponge, or compress covering the wound, with the perchloride or persulphate of iron, which, as a powerful astringent, when brought in contact with fresh blood, will immediately form a clot. Either of these preparations of iron poured into a wound, or the injection of a solution of perchloride of iron into the wound, not using force enough to infiltrate the tissues, is an excellent method of establishing a solid clot up to the very bleeding mouth of the injured vessel. These preparations of iron are also used in the form of powder, and are equally efficacious. A lump of ice placed upon the compress will act with equal vigor. A sponge or compress, tied on the bleeding wound, with or without the iron styptic, is all that the surgeon superintending the transportation of the wounded is expected to do. Unless the hemorrhage is very violent, threatening immediate destruction of life, the tourniquet is rarely required, All recent writers on military surgery recommend that field tourniquets be dispensed with, as they are generally a useless, and often, when carelessly used, a dangerous instrument, and our extensive experience has not advanced their utility. They are still issued in large numbers, and called for by army surgeons only because they are upon the supply table for field service; but very few of them are ever removed from the medical store-chest, where they remain as mementos of a former practice. Surgeons of large experience on many bloody battle-fields have never seen it necessary to apply them. The finger pressure of an intelligent assistant is better than any tourniquet ever made, and is a far preferable means of controlling excessive hemorrhage, which the compress and bandage may fail to check. The femoral artery, for any injury to its trunk or large branches, should be compressed in the groin where it runs over the pubic bone; the brachial, where it pulsates against the head of the humerus, as at this point its course is nearly subcutaneous. When the position of these main trunks are shown to any intelligent assistant, and he is made to recognize the throbbing of the artery, he will have no difficulty in keeping the vessel compressed during the transportation. Should the surgeon be doubtful of the exact position of the vessel or the intelligence of his assistant, the finger may be thrust into the depths of the wound and be applied directly to the seat of injury in the vessel, thus temporarily checking, and if sufficiently long continued, often permanently controlling, the bleeding.

Bruce A. Evans, M.D.
Control of Hemorrhage in Wounds
From: A Manual of Minor Surgery. John Packard, M.D.,
J.B. Lippincott & Co., Philadelphia 1863

The ligature, now so universally known as a means of arresting the current of blood through arteries, and sometimes through veins also, was first substituted for the cautery by the great French surgeon, Pare, in 1552. Various materials have from time to time been proposed for the making of ligatures, as well as for sutures; leaden wire, cat-gut, deer-skin thongs, and silken thread. "Saddler's silk" has perhaps, however, been more employed for the purpose than anything else; it may be varied in size according to that of the vessel to be secured, but should always be round and even, and. capable of withstanding a very firm pull. It should be well waxed for use.

A ligature may be applied either to the wounded portion of the artery, or at a point nearer the heart, the vessel being laid bare by an incision made for the purpose. In order to secure the end of an artery in a wound, a hook or tenaculum may be inserted in it, or it may be grasped with a pair of forceps; the forceps now made are generally provided with a wedge-shaped slide, which is pushed down through a perforated catch attached to the other blade, so as to ensure their hold. Some surgeons prefer the fenestrated forceps, or the catch-forceps of Liston, for this purpose. The (self-closing) spring-forceps ordinarily supplied in the army operating-cases has the advantage that the ligature may be drawn tight without any risk of the knot including the tip of the instrument; the vessel, once grasped, is securely held without the hand, and there is no slide, which is always liable to rust and become useless. When from necessity or choice the surgeon is without an assistant, he may simply allow the forceps or tenaculum to hang from the end of the vessel, or he may himself hold the latter instrument between his teeth, while his hands are engaged in applying the ligature. Generally this duty is entrusted to the assistant, the operator himself picking out the arteries with the tenaculum or forceps; the knot should always be made on that side of the vessel which is in view, and should be a very neat one, the hands being changed between the loops. An ordinary double or sailor's knot is most commonly used; the "surgeon's knot" is made when one end of the ligature is carried twice around the other in making the first tie. If the vessel to be secured is at the bottom of a deep wound, the operator pushes the knot down, as he makes it, with a forefinger on each end of the thread, rendered tense by the corresponding thumb and middle finger. One end of the ligature is cut off close, the other is allowed to hang out at the wound. When it is necessary to take up an artery in its continuity, it is exposed by an incision through the skin at the desired point, crossing the line of the vessel at a very acute angle; the successive layers of fascia, and the sheath of the artery, are in turn pinched up with a pair of forceps, nicked, and laid open on a grooved director; and finally the ligature is carried under the isolated vessel by means of a blunt needle with an eye near its point, and tied as in the former case.

The immediate effect of surrounding an artery with a tightly-drawn ligature is the division of its inner and middle coats, and the occlusion of its channel; the contained blood coagulates, and sooner or later the inner coat and this coagulum become consolidated together for some distance; the clot extends as far back as the next considerable branch which is given off, just as in the case of spontaneous cessation already mentioned.

We may generally look for the separation of ligatures from the fifth to the twelfth day after that of their application; it is due to the destructive ulceration of the vessel at the strictured point. If one or more large arteries are concerned, the threads placed about them should be very carefully handled, lest they come away too soon; it is as well to leave both ends of the ligature on such a vessel, tying them together so that they may be at once recognized among the single threads securing the smaller ones.

Bruce A. Evans, M.D.

Hospital Gangrene

Hospital gangrene is an apparently contagious affliction of a wound, characterized by initial intense, sharp, pricking pain and the appearance of a layer of ash-colored matter in the wound or ulcer base, which is firmly adherent and cannot be brushed or washed free. The granulation in the wound takes on a blue-red hue instead of a healthy pink. The edges of the wound become everted or undermined and are initially a livid, violet color, accompanied by a thin, watery, ash colored discharge. The surrounding area becomes swollen, reddened and firm. Progression occurs by daily enlargement, with mortification of the involved tissues to a gray, ash-colored slough. Untreated, it is fatal.

Prevention of spread requires no sharing of sponges or re-used dressings, &c, isolation of cases, and requiring assistants to dress the wounds of the gangrene patients last, and wash their hands between cases. The use of bromine or chlorine vapor as disinfectant treatments in the wards has been advocated.

Initially, the mortified tissue was treated with nitric acid and other caustics. Bromine solution has proven superior. This treatment usually requires use of chloroform due to the pain of the procedure, which involves the daily application of bromine solution throughout the wound following cleaning and drying the wound to remove debris from the previous treatment until heathy granulation tissue appears. This treatment, carefully followed, and appropriate prevention of spread has removed much to the previous terror of this disease.

Modern Perspective:

This extremely aggressive infection complicating wounds was a terror of the early-war hospitals.

It is difficult now to identify the responsible bacteria. What is now called "gas gangrene" is a specific infection that affects tissues without adequate circulation, and by clinical description is not the disease usually identified as hospital gangrene in the Civil War records. The speed of the spread of infection recalls modern descriptions to the Streptococcal "flesh eating" infection. Most likely, it represented an infection by multiple bacteria.

The contagious nature was recognized, and the precautions found to be effective in preventing its spread - including washing hands between patients, discarding wound cleaning materials, etc., could have come quite close to suggesting the germ theory of disease.

Without antibacterial agents, the only treatment found helpful was to literally destroy the involved tissues - along with the infectious agent - with caustic materials. This approach was benefited by the tendency of the disease to respect connective tissue divisions in the limb and remain superficial for much of it's early course. Nitric acid had been used with some success, but it is very difficult to get the acid to all the tissues in the depths of a wound, due to its rapid neutralization by tissue fluids. Bromine solution was found to work better, probably because it remained caustic even when diluted by tissue fluids and because its vapor, also caustic, would penetrated throughout the wound and remain active if it was kept in the would by "vapor dressings".

The conquest of hospital gangrene is an unrecognized achievement of Civil War Medicine.

Period Resource:

Gangrene — Collected From Various Medical Sources

General

The term "gangrene" is derived from the Greek for "I eat", referring to the erosive and tissue consuming nature of the affliction. The terms used include mortification, sphacelus, dry gangrene, moist gangrene, hospital gangrene, and gangrenous phagedema. Confusion due to the multiplicity of terms often idiosyncratically used leads to imprecise knowledge of occurrence of subtypes, but the overall incidence appears to be 1 per 1000 shot wounds, with a mortality of 46%, including deaths due to the wound itself or other complications.

Clinical Diagnosis

Dry gangrene: this is due to interruption of the blood supply, either traumatic or surgical. Often a sharp pain is felt at the onset, followed by painless progression of dry mortification of distal tissues characterized by blackening and shrinking, then dissolution. The treatment is early surgical resection above the border between the dead and the viable tissue.

Hospital gangrene: this is an apparently contagious affliction of a wound, characterized by initial intense, sharp, pricking pain and the appearance of a layer of ash-colored matter in the wound or ulcer base, which is firmly adherent and cannot be brushed or washed free. This usually occurs following a cessation of the normal healing and healthy granulation of the wound base, with appearance of punctate red spots in the wound and free bleeding with dressing changes. The granulation in the wound takes on a blue-red hue instead of a healthy pink. The edges of the wound become everted or undermined and are initially a livid, violet color, accompanied by a thin, watery, ash colored discharge. The surrounding area becomes swollen, reddened and firm. Progression occurs by daily enlargement, with mortification of the involved tissues to a gray, ash-colored slough and expansion usually limited to the skin and tissues down to the superficial fascia but occasionally involving the deep tissues and muscles. Sometimes but not invariably it is accompanied by an extremely offensive odor. Systemic symptoms include fever, coated tongue, sleepiness and malaise progressing to increasing prostration and death.

Treatment

Prevention: Relieve patient crowding; there is to be no sharing of sponges or re-used dressings, etc. Isolate cases of hospital gangrene, preferably in tents or well-ventilated places. Nurses should dress the wounds of the gangrene patients last, and wash their hands between cases. The use of bromine or chlorine vapor as disinfectant treatments in the wards has been advocated.

Treatment: Initially the mortified tissue was treated with nitric acid and other caustics. After mid war, increasing use of bromine as a caustic has been seen. The bromine solution is made up with one ounce of bromine, mixed with 160 grains of bromide of potassium and distilled water to 4 ounces.

Pans filled with one ounce of the prepared fluid can be placed throughout ward in sufficient numbers to cause a noticeable odor.

Treatment of Wound: This treatment usually requires use of chloroform due to the pain of the following procedure.

1. Clean and dry wound with absorbent cloth.
2. Trim sloughs with forceps and scissors to reduce thickness, then dry again
3. Apply bromine solution with stick or mop to saturate the slough; if overly thick inject into sloughs with needle. Solution must reach all recesses of the wound.
4. Follow with "vapor dressing": Dry lint placed over wound, followed by lint soaked in bromine solution, then more lint coated with simple cerate [simple salve], followed by oiled silk and bandage.
5. Repeat treatment every two hours as long as odor of mortification persists. Thereafter, use dressings soaked with dilute chlorinated soda.

The expected progress:

Day 2: surface firm, dark, and charred appearing

Day 3: dead portions begin to liquefy

Day 4: surface studded with healing granulations

Additional treatment is supportive and stimulating. Amputation of the involved part is the treatment of last resort and is occasionally successful.

Mortification of Wounds

The character of a wound as it progresses toward healing follows a progression. The discharge of pus - usually creamy and white - gradually diminishes. Healthy pink granulation tissue in evident within the wound, filling in from the depths of the wound with time. Evidence of inflammation wanes, with decreased swelling and redness of the tissues preceding the filling in of the wound with healthy granulation tissue as it heals.

A turn for the worse in the healing process may occur at the very start, or interrupt an apparently favorable course to that point. The discharge of pus increases, becoming more thin and watery, and often foul-smelling. The tissues within the wound become softened, dark, and may slough in pieces. A hectic fever often appears, and the patient begins to sink, with emaciation, a weak thready pulse, and finally a low muttering delirium, coma, and death. Alternatively, the wound may develop the characteristics of hospital gangrene or erysipelas, or the patient may expire quickly from evident pyemia. Disinfectants applied to the wound are of little help, although they may reduce the foulness of the wound that makes caring for the patient obnoxious. Caustics to change the character of the wound also seem of little benefit in modifying the course, with the exception of bromine used early in hospital gangrene.

Modern Perspective:

"Mortification" was either the persistence and progression of an initial wound infection, or the occurrence of a new infection in a healing wound. In the pre-antisepsis era, such infection could not be prevented, and without antibiotics, could not be effectively treated when they occurred. The changing character

of the pus discharge from creamy, white - "laudable" - pus to a foul smelling, watery discharge signaled a secondary infection with a more deadly, aggressive bacteria such as clostridium or pseudomonas. Without defense, this was a lethal change.

Antiseptics were used on mortifying wounds, but at that point their rather weak antibacterial potency was of little benefit against an established infection. Although antiseptics were used in hospitals to attempt to prevent contagion, they were placed in pans throughout the area - including chlorine and bromine - in the hope the vapors would be of preventative benefit. The use of disinfectants such as carbolic acid applied to the skin before infection occurred was not known until Lister's publications beginning in 1867.

Pyemia

Pyemia may complicate any wound at any point in its course. Wounds complicated by fractures are the most susceptible. The affliction begins with shaking chills accompanied by an increased fever.

With great speed, the patient becomes prostrate, sinking quickly through delirium, coma, and death, often within hours. Treatment is advocated with tonics and stimulants, and a supportive diet but is uniformly ineffective.

Modern Perspective:

Pyemia (pus in the blood, "blood poisoning") was a feared complication of any wound, and uniformly fatal.

It represents what we now recognize as sepsis, the release into the bloodstream of massive numbers of pathogenic bacteria. Treatment of sepsis can still be challenging in the antibiotic era, although that challenge is usually due to antibiotic resistance.

Given that every wound was infected, the occurrence of sepsis is unsurprising. It was most likely to complicate wounds where localized infection, poor pus drainage, and rich blood supply came together. That is the reason, for example, for the high mortality of shot fractures involving joints, and the basis for such a fracture indicating the need for amputation.

Tetanus

The incidence is 2 per 1000 wounds, with a disproportionate involvement in lower extremity wounds. Over 90% of the cases are fatal, and those that survive are milder from onset and of later onset. In some of the surviving cases the diagnosis is to be doubted.

The cause is uncertain, but possibilities include heat exposure, cold and damp exposure, neglect of thorough wound cleaning, and damage to nerves during probing of wounds.

The symptoms begin with typical neck and mouth pain and stiffness, leading to forcible closure of the mouth due to jaw muscle spasms (trismus). This is followed by spread of painful muscle spasms throughout the body, often triggered by touch or other stimuli. Finally, exhaustion and death supervene.

Tetanus may be more common in hospitals located in barns and other multi-use buildings than in tents or open areas. The reason is unknown.

Usual treatments attempted include chloroform (Pannier #16), ether, opiates, stimulants, external irritants, and fomentations (application of clothes soaked in hot water or medicated decoction).

Specific internal medications include bromide of potassium, tincture of aconite (Pannier #), belladonna, Hoffman's anodyne (Pannier #20), camphor, castor oil, turpentine (Pannier #26), and croton oil.

External treatments include external blisters, emollients, turpentine (Pannier #26), ice, creosote (Pannier #46), warm baths, bagged ice and salt. The mere number of medications and treatments attempted speaks to the futility of treatment in these cases.

Modern Perspective;

The symptoms of tetanus are caused by a toxin to nerves produced by a bacterium called Clostridium tetani. This bacterium forms spores which are resistant to heat and drying; the spores are ubiquitous, and are frequently found in animal dung, dirt, and dust. When gaining entry to man through a skin break, the bacteria begin to reproduce in areas with little blood flow, producing toxin which spreads through the body, being taken up by nerve endings. The toxin is taken up primarily in inhibitory neurons, and as they are inactivated, the typical spasms of tetanus occur. The action of the toxin is irreversible, so prevention prior to symptoms by immunization against the toxin is necessary.

Even today, a symptomatic case of tetanus is often fatal.

Categorization of Medications by Action

Period pharmacology texts categorized medications by their presumed primary action. As the precise mechanisms of action were unknown, these actions were determined either by observable effects or, in some cases, by theoretical considerations.

Bear in mind that without the ability to know disease mechanisms, the physicians were treating symptoms and attempting to return the observable changes towards the normal state. Stimulants and sedatives were prescribed based on the character of the disease in question. When that was predominantly "dynamic" – fever, flushing, forceful and rapid pulse, visible inflammation, and active delirium – the disease process was considered "phlogistic" and sedation (most often accompanied by drugs affecting function such as cathartics, emetics, etc., which were felt to deplete the system of excess excitement) was the treatment of choice. The use of trying to draw off the abnormal inflammation by producing a local irritation – such as with cupping or irritative skin plasters - was based on the theory that the system could only sustain a certain amount of inflammation at a time. This would be accompanied also by a scanty, "low" diet, as in the old saying "starve a fever".

When the character of the disease was, on the other hand, exhibited weakness, prostration, weak pulse, paleness, and low or "muttering" delirium the disease process was considered "adynamic" or "putrid" and was best treated by stimulant therapy and robust, "high" diet rich in easily digestible nutrients including beef tea, milk punch, and eggs. "Feed a cold."

These principles were tempered by experience in two ways.

Some diseases were known to have an early "dynamic" appearance but rapidly and inexorably progress to an adynamic or putrid state so depletion and sedation at the onset were avoided.

A (very) few diseases had empirically known "specific" treatment such as quinine products for true intermittent fever (malaria) and colchicine for gout. This knowledge trumped theory.

The material presented here is abstracted from period medical and pharmacology texts. Modern perspectives may be consulted in the sections on specific diseases and specific medications.

Affecting Function

Medications affecting function are mostly used to increase one or more of the physiologic secretions, or discharges from the body. The utility of such treatment can be characterized as follows:

- To restore natural secretion when decreased by torpor or vascular insufficiency
- To augment natural secretion to decrease circulating fluid
- To augment natural secretion to promote absorption (dropsy)
- To augment natural secretion of a part, to decrease that of another part
- To augment natural secretion of an organ, to relieve determinants of blood to another where inflammation is taking place (e.g., evacuants in brain disease)
- To promote secretion to favor subsidence of disease whose natural termination is accompanied (perhaps caused) by increased secretion
- To produce exhaustion as anti-phlogisitics (in diseases characterized by excess action)

Affecting Function – Cathartics

Cathartics are medicines which provoke bowel movements. The utility of this function in disease includes:

- To evacuate the contents of the bowels and to relieve symptoms caused by retained contents such as retained feculent matter, undigested food, and morbid secretions.
- To promote secretion and exhalation when secretion is decreased (torpid affections), to clean the blood of morbid agents which ought to have been excreted by other routes, to decrease circulatory volume for relief of plethora and congestion, to promote absorption, to substitute for other decreased secretion, and for relief of inflammation through local and systemic depletion.
- To promote secretion of the liver and pancreas for congestion or torpor of the portal system (liver-bowel circulation).
- To stimulate or excite the muscles of the alimentary canal for torpor.
- To affect nearby organs on principle of revulsion (drawing inflammation away from one organ by irritating another).

Classes of cathartics and examples of their use include:
- Laxatives (mild cathartics): tamarind, prunes, bitartrate of potash, fixed oils (castor oil, olive oil)
- Saline, antiphlogistic, or cooling cathartics: the neutral salts as used for diaphoretics, but for this function are used in concentrations greater than in the blood.

- Milder acrid cathartics: senna, rhubarb, aloes. These are acrids and stimulants, but not enough to cause inflammation of the stomach and bowels.
- Senna: active but not overly irritant
- Rhubarb: when tonic properties needed (for relaxed and debilitated condition of alimentary tract)
- Drastic cathartics: jalap, croton, colocynth

These are used for torpid conditions of bowels, as hydrogogues (to draw water away from the body) in dropsy, and as counter-irritants in brain disease. (not in inflammatory or irritated bowel disease due to their irritating effect on the bowels and stomach).

Mercurials: these are alterative purgatives and appear to be useful to promote hepatic function as purges. They are, however, somewhat uncertain in cathartic action, so use combined with or followed by other more certain purges is appropriate.

Pannier Medications of this class:

#31 Pilulae Cartharticae Compositae
#32 Pills of Ext. Colycin. Comp. and Ipecac
#41 Pilulae Hydrargyri
#6 Hydrargyri Chloridium Mite
#26 Oleum Terebinthinae

Affecting Function – Emetics

Emetics are medicines which provoke vomiting. The effect of these medications may be indicated by a description of therapeutic vomiting:

Within 20-30 minutes, a sense of unease and nausea begins and intensifies. The pulse becomes small, feeble, and irregular. The face and lips become pale. Then begins an unpleasant sense of relaxation, faintness and coldness of the whole system. Saliva begins to flow copiously, the eyes lose luster, and the whole countenance is dejected. With the onset of vomiting, the pulse becomes frequent and full, there is an increased temperature, and sweat breaks out. Vomiting is then accompanied by violent straining, with swollen and discolored face, engorged veins, tears bursting from eyes, and occasional involuntary expulsion of urine and feces with straining.

This description makes clear the powerful forces unleashed by these medications, which some feel serve an important revulsive function, drawing inflammation away from internal organs.

Their uses in disease include:

- To evacuate stomach (expelling poisons or undigested food)
- For this use, generally the mildest of these drugs is used, such as ipecac.
- For poisons, use zinc sulphate or copper sulphate, due to faster action and less nausea.
- To excite nausea and thereby depress vascular and muscular systems in sthenic disease: tartar emetic in

full emetic doses may be used in "strong subjects" for this use.
- To reduce vascular action in some hemorrhages, in inflammatory fever, acute inflammation of lungs, testicles, mammae, bronchial tubes, skin, and joints. Note, however, that due to direct irritation of the stomach and bowels by these drugs, they are unsafe in inflammation of the alimentary canal.
- To promote secretion and excretion in hepatic disease (probably by increasing bile and pancreatic secretion and secretion by gastric mucosa), and in inflammation of the bronchial tubes, larynx and throat (probably by local increased secretion).

Pannier Medications of this class:

#49 Extractum Ipecacuahnae
#52 Zinci Sulphas
#32 Pills of Ext. Colycin. Comp. and Ipecac
#18 Syrupus Scillae
#5 Antimonii et Potass

Affecting Function – Diuretics

Diuretics are medicines which increase urination. The uses in the disease state include:
- Restore kidney action in disease characterized by diminished urine
- Promote absorption in dropsy
- Augment elimination of water to keep minerals in bladder in solution in stone disease
- Relieve inflammation (especially salines/neutral salts)
- Many diuretic medications have other useful properties, and are also represented elsewhere in this classification.

Pannier Medications of this class:
#12 Spiritus Aetheris Nitrici
#36 Potassae Bicarbonas
#50 Tinctura Ferri Chloridi
#11 Spiritus Frumenti
#35 Potassae Chloras
#4 Iodinum
#26 Oleum Terebinthinae
#18 Syrupus Scillae

Affecting Function – Diaphoretics

Diaphoretics are medicines which increase perspiration. As a class, these medications are uncertain in their action of producing sweating and, truthfully, of uncertain benefit to the patient, and success is attained only in certain body states.

The diaphoretic action is promoted by use of diluents (increased water intake), keeping the skin warm, and with use at bedtime. They are not to be used with diuretics, as diuretics check the action of diaphoretics.

Uses of diaphoretics in disease include:

- Restore sweating when checked by cold to relieve ill effects (catching cold)
- Promote subsidence of disease which naturally terminates with sweat or with exanthematous eruptions (simple continued fever, exanthemata -diseases associated with skin rash like measles, small pox, etc.- intermittents)
- Promote determination (strong direction to a given point) to the skin in maladies associated with cold skin and internal inflammation, to reduce the internal inflammation.
- To antagonize other secretions that are excessive due to disease action, such as excessive urination or diarrhea (i.e., with opium, which will also directly antagonize these symptoms)

- To substitute perspiration as pathway for water excretion for other secretions reduced by disease action (i.e., in dropsy due to granular degeneration of the kidney)

Classes of Diaphoretics and their suggested uses include:

- Aqueous diuretics: water, etc.
- Alkaline salts and neutral salines: ammonium acetate and ammonium citrate, alkaline citrates/tartrates, sal ammoniac, nitrate of potash. These are especially useful for fevers
- Antimonial (i.e., tartar emetic): this is useful for febrile or inflammatory cases, and is preferred to opium if inflammation or congestion of brain is present due to the stimulation of the brain caused by opium.
- Opiates: these are useful, especially as Dover's Powders, when no brain inflammation is present and especially if an anodyne is needed (pain relief) or with rheumatism. It is preferred to antimony if bowels irritable due to the irritating effect on the bowels of antimony, and the quieting effect of opium.
- Oleaginous and resinous: camphor, sassafras (active oil)
- Alcohol
- Ipecac: this medication may not have much of this activity as has been supposed.

Pannier Medications of this class:
#12 Spiritus Aetheris Nitrici
#4 Iodinum
#5 Antimonii et Potas. Tartras
#11 Spiritus Frumenti

#49 Extractum Ipecacuahnae
#33 Pills of Pulv. Ipecac et Opii
#39 Liquor Morphae Sulphas
#32 Pills of Ext. Colycin. Comp. and Ipecac

Affecting Function – Expectorants

Expectorants are medicines which promote coughing. They are used exclusively for lung problems. Two main classes are used:

- Emollient and nauseating properties for acute bronchial irritations: tartar emetic and ipecac
- Stimulating expectorants are of use for chronic lung disease, including seneka, especially in the latter stages of acute bronchitis, and "fetid gums," such as garlic, for chronic bronchitis.

Pannier Medications of this class:
  #32 Pills of Ext. Colycin. Comp. and Ipecac
  #5 Antimonii et Potas. Tartras
  #49 Extractum Ipecacuahnae
  #37 Potassii Iodium

Stimulants – Astringents

Astringents cause a non-muscular contraction of tissue through a mechanism which is unknown. The effect is both local and, to some extent, systemic, probably more by the mechanism of sympathy (i.e., organ to organ effect of the autonomic nerves) than by absorption and distribution of the drug by the blood.

Secondary effects include narrowing of the blood vessels and ducts, decreased secretion, exhalation, and absorption by the surface treated, constipation, increased firmness of the pulse, and increased coagulability of the blood. In excess, these drugs are often irritating or damaging.

Indications for their use include morbid discharges or hemorrhages, morbid relaxation of tissues, and early stages of inflammation where direct application of the drug to the involved area is possible.

Astringents decrease morbid secretions by contracting the pores in blood vessels which create the secretions. Examples of such use include (external) treatment of: chronic coryza(nasal discharge), purulent ophthalmia (pus discharge from the eyes), gonorrhea, and rectal discharge. These drugs should be used with great caution if at all if the morbid secretion is caused by – and in fact serves to relieve - a plethora (area of vascular congestion), an area of active inflammation, or the presence of noxious matter, since blocking the outflow without treating the cause would cause great harm. In these cases, use after appropriate depletion treatment is possible, when the discharge itself is a danger, as in dysentery.

Astringents treat the morbid relaxation of tissues that is often associated with a morbid discharge, especially when the disorder is chronic (long standing). Examples include convalescence from febrile and other acute diseases, such as the chronic inflammation of the stomach and bowels when the acute stage of dysentery is past and the blood and lymph vessels are passively distended or ulcerations persist. External use examples include the treatment of hemorrhoids, prolapsed anus, and indolent, flabby skin ulcers.

These agents are useful as primary anti-inflammation treatment only in cases of external inflammation when sufficient dose can be applied to decrease the blood supply supporting the inflammation. Examples include inflammation in the mouth or the tonsilar area, inflammation in the rectum, in the skin, or in the mucous membranes of the genito-urinary system.

Representatives include Tannic Acid, Alum, and Acetate of Lead.

Note that lead poisoning is dangerous and must be watched for with any substantial or chronic use. Toxic symptoms of lead include, progressively:

- prodrome: lead/blue or slate/blue line on gum margins, especially incisors; bluish-red tint to gums; teeth stained brown, especially lowers; peculiar taste and breath odor; skin and sclera 'earthy-yellow' hue
- lead colic (severe, cramping abdominal pain)
- arthralgias (joint pains)
- paralysis of arms, legs
- disease of encephalon (encephalopathy, delirium, coma)

Pannier Medications of this class:
#51 Plumbi Acetas
#44 Alumen

#43 Acidum Tannicum
#29 Liquor Ferri Perisulphatus

Stimulants – Diffuseable

These stimulants act quickly and vigorously, but for a shorter time than the permanent stimulants. Their force of action is generally greater than the permanent stimulants. They also are characterized by a more profound depression after the action has waned than permanent agents.

They are indicated in cases of considerable and, especially, sudden or acute prostration, when the action of tonics or diet would be too slow. Care must be taken that the apparent prostration is not due to inflammation of a deep organ requiring depletion rather than stimulation.

Stimulation can be used with caution to help maintain heart action and pulse in a patient requiring vigorous depletion to treat a severe internal congestion. In such cases, the stimulation must be ended before reaction sets in, or the inflammation may be worsened. This consideration mandates the use of stimulants whose effect may be quickly ended, such as ammonia, heat, ether, or external stimulation. Similar issues arise with treatment of the depression of the system after a brain concussion, any severe injury, surgery, or during the cold stage of a severe febrile illness. In all these cases, avoidance of inappropriate intensity or length of stimulation is critical to prevent danger to the patient.

Debility in the setting of an acute febrile disease can be treated with vigorous stimulation with little fear of reaction. In low or typhoid fever, stimulation is necessary to sustain life, and accompanying inflammation should be treated cautiously with cups, leeches, fomentations, blisters, etc.

An initially inflammatory disease which takes a depraved turn to debility and poisoned blood, such as is often seen with typhous pneumonia, typhous dysentery, malignant sore throat, smallpox, and erysipelas, should be approached with the same concern for appropriate stimulation and gentle depletion only as necessary, as should inflammatory disease in a previously debilitated patient (enfeebled by disease, bad living, or drunkenness).

Heat

Heat is a universal stimulant, acting upon all tissues and organs.

Arterial Stimulants

Arterial stimulants generate warmth and heat, increase the frequency and the force of the pulse, and increase the surface temperature of the body. They are used externally and internally. These are especially good for treatment of the collapse associated with severe injury, since they do not affect the brain. They should not be used in cases of gastric inflammation, due to local irritation.

Representatives include Capsicum, Cayenne Pepper, Oil of Turpentine, and Carbonate of Ammonia

Pannier Medications of this class:

#1 Capsici Pulvis
#30 Spiritus Ammoniae Aromaticus
#26 Oleum Terebinthinae
#24 Extract Zingiberis Fluidum
#19 Liquor Ammoniae

Nervous Stimulants

Nervous stimulants stimulate the nervous system generally, without specifically acting on the brain. Most also have arterial stimulation qualities as an incidental effect. Many are aromatic, and are disagreeable in odor or taste.

These agents are indicated in for both overaction (paradoxically, perhaps due to "equalizing excitement" by drawing excess action from diseased to non-diseased areas stimulated by the drug) and depression of nervous function, if functional and not due to inflammation or congestion best treated with depletion or other antiphlogisitc treatments. There is danger of repeated doses losing effect through habituation.

These agents are contraindicated in sthenic disease with inflammation and fever, especially when the seat of inflammation is in the nervous centers themselves. They also don't work in severe nervous diseases deeply placed in the brain or spinal centers, such as apoplexy, epilepsy, insanity, palsy, tetanus, or coma.

Specific indications include:

- Morbid excitability of nervous centers.
- Spasmodic afflictions, such as muscle cramps, spasms of the stomach, bowels, or bladder, clonic spasms or convulsions, asthma, and hiccoughs.
- Irregular movements of voluntary muscles such as restlessness, ties, crying, sobbing, or hyperventilation.
- Disordered sensation such as malaise, weariness, itching, tingling, neuraligic pains, headache, dizziness, head fullness, etc.

- Mental disorders such as emotional perversions, hypochondriasis, obstinate wakefulness, nightmares, etc..
- Derangements of organic functions such as palpitations, fainting, nausea, vomiting, flatulence, dyspnea, borborygmi (rumbling of bowels), excessive diruresis, etc., when not due to inflammation or organic disease. When these symptoms are due to hysteria the agents help greatly. When due to nervous rheumatism, some help may be expected.

Representatives include Castor Oil, Valerian, Garlic, Coffee, and Tea

Pannier Medications of this class:

#23 Extract Valerianae Fluidum
#8 Extract of Coffee
#10 Tea, Black

Cerebral Stimulants

Also known as the stimulant narcotics, these agents add to a stimulant effect on the circulation and the nervous system a peculiar power over the special functions of the brain, leading all the way to stupor and delirium. Other than this common description, these agents vary widely in degree of stimulant power, degree of cerebral specificity, manner of cerebral effect, and the effects on other organs.

Keep in mind that cerebral sedatives and stimulants may have similar effects. Opium (a stimulant) and aconite (a sedative) will both cause coma in excess, but only the sedative is indicated in active congestion of the brain, while the stimulant will cause harm. Similarly, chloroform (a sedative) and ether (a stimulant) will both cause insensibility.

The cerebral stimulants generally have the following effects:

- Excite the stomach
- Increase heart action
- Pervert the sensorial functions, causing intoxication and delirium, followed
- by decreased sensorial function leading to drowsiness and stupor
- Following a variable period of stimulation, there is a compensatory period of depression, coming on after from 1-12 hours of stimulation. Poisonous doses
- cause death by asphyxia (suffocation). These agents tend to lose effect by repetition.

Indications are often specific to the drug, but a few general comments can be made:

- Used for general stimulation if there is no active congestion or inflammation of the brain.
- Can be used for relief of pain (anodyne function), spasm (antispasmodic function), and nervous irritation (narcotic function), and in the production of sleep (soporific or hypnotic function).

Representatives include alcohol, ether, camphor, opium, belladonna

Pannier Medications of this class:

#20 Spiritus Aetheris Compositus

#28 Tinctura Opii Camphorata
#21 Tinctura Opii
#42 Pilulae Opii
#13 Alcohol Fortius
#33 Pills of Pulv. Ipecac et Opii
#40 Pills of Camphor and Opium

Stimulants – Tonics

Tonics increase the vital actions moderately, with a slow onset and a somewhat prolonged time of action. Actions include:

- promote appetite
- invigorate digestion
- increase pulse fullness, strength, and perhaps rate
- increase body temperature
- may increase various secretions
- increase the firmness of the muscles
- may have some effect on the nervous centers, especially the <u>organic</u> functions

These actions elevate the functions towards but not above levels reached in a state of natural health. Depression of these functions may follow a prolonged course of stimulation with tonics. There is danger of overstimulation leading to increased inflammation by treatment with tonics if some organs are the seats of chronic inflammation with increased blood flow and congestion.

Mechanisms of action of these drugs include acting on digestive tract to increase nutrition, acting directly on the blood to increase its quality, or, in the majority, acting directly on the target tissues.

These drugs are of great value in conditions of depressed and <u>torpid</u> function and debility.

Representatives of this class of drugs:

- Animal origin substances including Cod-Liver Oil
- Vegetable substances including the simple bitters, peculiar property bitters such as Peruvian Bark, Sulphate of Quinia,

and Chamomile, and aromatics such as Cloves, Nutmeg, Peppermint, and Ginger
- Mineral substances such as the mineral acids, including sulphuric acid, nitric acid, and muriatic acid, metallic substances such as silver nitrate, copper sulphate, sulphate of zinc, and reconstructive mineral tonics including various iron compounds

Pannier Medications of this class:

24 Extract Zingiberis Fluidum
29 Liquor Ferri Perisulphatus
22 Tinctura Cinchonas Fluidum
34 Pilulae Quiniae Sulphatis
50 Tinctura Ferri Chloridi

Sedatives – General

Sedatives form the basis of a depletion therapy for sthenic diseases (characterized by an excess of organism and tissue excitement; often associated with fever, inflammation, flushing, and increased heart action) through their action on tissue, vascular, and organ excitement.

General sedatives, by direct action, depress the vital actions. The effect is universal, on all organs and systems.

COLD may be used to treat such problems as vascular excitement ((e.g., cold compresses for congestion of brain), nervous excitement (e.g. cold baths for tetanus, cold compresses to epigastric area for stomach spasms), abnormal increase in body temperature (e.g. spraying with cold water for fever), or to decrease sensitivity to pain (e.g. use of ice for neuralgic pains). When using cold, care should be taken that the remedy is applied steadily and long enough that the object is accomplished. If used intermittently or for too short a time, reaction may occur (rebound of suppressed overactivity) resulting in greater injury than if the treatment had not been used. It is therefore appropriate for superficial and fixed inflammation, rather than for a manifestation of a severe and constitutional disorder such as rheumatism or gout, for which a more sustained and systemic remedy should be used.

WATER is a useful sedative.

In inflammation and vascular irritation, it is fruitfully used as an adjunctive depleting therapy. Local baths, cataplasms, and fomentations are useful for external disorders. It is used as an emollient cataplasm for furuncles (boils), glandular swellings, and inflamed joints after local depletion. In erysipelatous and erythematous affections, water is used in the form of demulcent liquids applied with soft linen compresses.

Water is also helpful for internal inflammation. For inflammation of the abdominal and pelvic viscera, in the form of fomentations, or better, large cataplasms covering the whole of the external parts corresponding to the inflamed organ. Gastritis, enteritis, dysentery, peritonitis, hepatitis, and nephritis are all appropriately treated in this fashion. A warm bath, in addition, is often helpful.

Water is less useful in idiopathic fevers than in the phlegmasiae (an older term for the sthenic diseases), but it is most advantageously used in nervous diseases such as spasmodic and convulsive afflictions including colic, strangulated hernia, stomach spasms, gall duct spasm, bladder spasms, and even tetanus. It is also useful in all forms of hysteria.

Sedatives – Depleting

Sedatives form the basis of a depletion therapy for sthenic diseases (characterized by an excess of organism and tissue excitement; often associated with fever, inflammation, flushing, and increased heart action) through their action on tissue, vascular, and organ excitement.

Direct depletion is accomplished mainly by **BLEEDING**, and also by increasing the various sections (the latter discussed under local actions later). Since blood sustains and supports all functions, bleeding is a general sedative. Bleeding sequentially reduces the force and fullness of the pulse, leading to paleness, then to decreased temperature, and eventually to loss of force of the pulse and syncope (fainting).

If too much blood is removed (more than 17-20 oz. in a basically healthy man), the reaction can damage the system as centers struggle to increase the blood supply leading to violent palpitations of the heart, excessive rate of the pulse, and eventually dyspnea (shortness of breath), headache, convulsions, and delirium - all caused by the attempt to summon excess blood to centers threatened by the systemic loss of blood. For this reason, bleeding to syncope for the purpose of depletion is not indicated.

Bleeding may be performed generally with opening of a vein or artery, or locally with scarification (superficial cuts from a knife or an apparatus designed to produce an number of small superficial cuts at one time), wet or dry cupping, or with leeches.

Indications are serious inflammation, usually acute rather than chronic, and especially in the early stages. Even when indicated, use is limited by the need to preserve the vital functions of the blood necessary to restore health by resolving abnormal consolidation of tissue (as in the lung in pneumonia), to resolve abnormal serous or fibrin exudates (as in the bowel in severe dysentery), or to support healing suppuration (pus formation) or the healing of ulcers.

Indirect depletion can be accomplished through manipulations of **DIET**, affecting the system's nutrition. This may be accomplished through abstinence from food, a decreased amount of food, or the use of a "low" diet. The nutritive value of the diet can be adjusted in several gradations appropriate to various levels of need for depletion therapy. The lowest diet is bland and consists of vegetable elements only. The diet consists of gums, starches, and sugars, often in a watery solution or infusions. The most commonly used are gum arabic, slippery elm bark, arrowroot, barley water, rice water, refined sugar, and molasses. The next step up involves the inclusion of more nutritive nitrogenous vegetable substances, including albumen, gluten, and vegetable fixed oils. These can be supplied in cornmeal or oatmeal gruel, boiled rice, toasted wheat bread and wheat crackers. Further elevation of the diet involves inclusion of milk. The final elevation of the diet, yet short of a normal full diet, involves the inclusion of boiled meats.

ARTERIAL sedatives decrease the force of the circulation by their immediate action rather than indirectly by depletion, and are without a direct effect on the nervous system. Paradoxically, these substances may be locally irritating.

They are useful in all diseases with excess arterial excitement in the setting of a sthenic state. Examples are inflammation, high vascular irritation, and fever characterized by vigorous action. For such problems, the antimonials such as tartar emetic (generally doses below those producing vomiting) are appropriate. Only the weakest drugs of this class (i.e., the neutral salts-neutral mixture, effervescent draught, or citric acid) should be used for fever or vascular excitement in putrid or low diseases such as typhoid fever or phthisis (tuberculosis).

Pannier Medications of this class:

#5 Antimonii et Potas. Tartras

NERVOUS sedatives, reduce nervous power by direct effect without a pronounced effect on cerebral functions, and secondarily reduce the circulation.

These drugs are indicated both in nervous irritation and in excessive heart action, especially when both are present. Since they are not as effective for inflammation as the arterial sedatives, they are not first line antiphlogistic drugs.

Pannier Medications of this class:

#47 Extractum Aconti Radicis Fluidum

#48 Extractum Colchici Seminis Fluidum

CEREBRAL sedatives directly depress cerebral as well as spinal functions, with indirect effects on the circulation and the heart. By definition, they profoundly affect consciousness, intellect, and the emotions.

Prussic acid (hydrocyanic acid) is useful in allaying nervous irritation, especially involving the heart action, such as palpitations and irregularity of the heartbeat.

Chloroform is useful for:

- Relieving and preventing pain, such as angina pectoris or neuralgic pain
- Relaxing spasm, as when inhaled for asthma
- Promoting sleep, especially in delirium tremens
- Calming nervous irritation
- Hysteria
- As a surgical anesthetic

Pannier Medications of this class:

#16 Chloroformum Purificatum

Alteratives

Alteratives are medications that, without elevating or depressing vital actions, produce changes in organization or function. The effects are usually unappreciable in health. The nature of the effect is usually unknown, and is evident only by the beneficial effect on disease. This benefit, therefore, has usually been discovered empirically.

The precise mechanisms of action are unknown, but some possibilities include:

- Modify condition of the blood, such as mercury "poisoning" the fibrin in blood preventing coagulation, or alkalis causing the same effect by making fibrin more soluble.
- Modify the state of solid tissues
- Neutralize, decompose, or eliminate some noxious agent, such as mercury curing syphilis by destroying the contagious element, colchicum curing gout by eliminating uric acid and urea through the kidneys, and iodide of potassium dislodging lead from the tissues into the blood to cure lead poisoning.

Each drug in this class has unique action and they must be considered
individually:

- Mercury is felt to stimulate and regulate hepatic function, and is thus good for hepatic disorders such as torpor, decreased bile, jaundice and clay-colored stools, or for benefit to abdominal organs by depletion from the portal circulation as for melena (blood in the stools).

- Mercury is no longer given for its effect on increasing salivation, and thus should not be given in doses larger than those causing an initial increase in saliva.
- Mercury is given to stimulate secretions in febrile disease characterized by dry skin and mouth, scanty urine, and constipation, such as the second stage of typhoid. Mercury (with opium) is helpful in bilious colic.
- Mercury promotes resolution and dispersion of chronic indurations (swellings)
- Mercury may work by promoting a "revolutionizing" effect, promoting disintegration of diseased tissues, and allowing natural recovery to occur. As such, it may be especially useful to check 'effusion' and promote removal of lymph already deposited by inflammation. It should not be used in chronic disease, and, as it is not a powerful antiphlogistic, it should not be used in the active, early phase of sthenic disease (regular depletion treatment- including perhaps tartar emetic - should be used first).
- Mercury is appropriate for bilious remittent fever, yellow fever, and the second stage of typhoid.
- Arsenic is useful as an antiperiodic (after quinia), for chronic cutaneous eruptions such as psoriasis and leprosy, and chronic eczema and impetigo.
- Iodine is specific for goiter, and is useful in other tumefactions (swellings) such as scrofula. It is also helpful in chronic and neuralgic rheumatism, and in lead and possibly mercury poisoning.
- Chlorine vapor is helpful in chronic bronchitis, for foul breath with purulent expectoration, and to correct fetid exhalations. Chlorine water is useful internally for febrile disease and topically for bites of mad dogs.

Pannier Medications of this class:

#41 Pilulae Hydrargyri
#6 Hydrargyri Chloridium Mite
#<u>4 Iodinium</u> – iodine
   <u>Hydrargyri</u> <u>unguent.</u> <u>nit</u>. - ointment of nitrate of mercury

Affecting Skin Structure for Local Effect

Topical medications are often used to disrupt the organization of the skin to various degrees. These medications are generally used to inflame or irritate the skin, for counter-irritation effect in inflammatory processes. When applied to skin overlying the affected organ, they serve to draw away inflammation from that organ. The medications are characterized by the degree to which they disrupt the organization of the tissue to which they are applied (almost always the skin).

Rubefacients

These medications cause redness of the skin only. Representatives include mustard (nigra-black, alba-white), zingifer (ginger root), capsicum (pepper), and turpentine.

Pannier Medications of this class:
　#1 Capsici Pulvis
　#26 Oleum Terebinthinae
　#19 Liquor Ammoniae

Epispastics

These medications cause mild to moderate blistering of the skin with formation of serous exudate (watery discharge). Representatives include cantherides (spanish fly) and croton oil.

Pannier Medications of this class:
#46 Creasotum

#1 Capsici Pulvis<u>Ceratum</u>

Escharotics

These medications cause damage well into the dermis, resulting is crops of pustules and sloughing away of the skin surface. Escharotics are used specifically to destroy unwanted tissue, in order to remove excresences or <u>morbid</u> growths, to open abcesses, or to provoke a draining wound for counter-irritative or <u>revulsive</u> purposes. Medications for this use include sulfuric acid, nitric acid, solid potassium, zinc chloride, and antimony terchloride.

Somewhat weaker agents than the forgoing are used to promote scarring and healing of ulcers, or stopping hemorrhage from numerous small blood vessels, including copper nitrate or silver nitrate.

Pannier Medications of this class:
#2 Argenti Nitras
#3 Argenti Nitras Fusus

Demulcents

These are bland, non-irritating substances which confer upon water, when place in solution, a quality of adhesiveness or viscosity. They generally consist of gummy, farinaceous, or saccharine substances.
Effects are mediated by:

- All<u>ow</u>ing inflamed surfaces to regain their natural moist quality, necessary to their proper function

- Direct reduction of the effect of the irritating cause
- Examples of these substances and their use include:
- Gum arabic held in the mouth for cough or tonsillar inflammation
- Flax seed infusion for catarrh or dysentery
- Sassafras pith infusions in the eye for ophthalmia
- Solid molasses held in the mouth for cough
- Glycerin externally for irritative cutaneous eruptions such as herpes, eczema, and psoriasis

Pannier Medications of this class:

#15 Sugar, White

Emollients

Emollients are bland and non-irritating substances which can be formed into a soft, slightly adhesive mass that when applied to the skin softens and relaxes its tissues. Unlike demulcents, these are used exclusively externally. They are mainly useful for superficial inflammation and vascular irritation, hastening cure by their sedative effect, and encouraging the formation of abscesses and put when the inflammation has progressed further, hastening ultimate healing.
Flaxseed meal, bread and milk, ground slippery-elm bark, and oatmeal are examples of substances used in this fashion.

Pannier Medications of this class:
#27 Glycerina
#25 Oleum Olivae
#17 Liniment

Diluents

Cool water-based drinks act as diluents throughout the system. They dilute the contents of the stomach and bowels, dilute the blood fol<u>low</u>ing absorption, and dilute the various excretions of the body when eliminated, including the urine and the sweat. They are thus useful in inflammatory or irritative processes of any of the surfaces involved in these transformations, including those in which the diluted liquid itself is irritating.

- Stomach (gastritis)
- Blood vessels (fever with hot skin and thirst)
- Urinary system (kidney: nephritis, urinary bladder: cystitis, ureathra: ureathritis)

Best administered cool or cold, the exact drink should be tailored to the
patient's taste, and possibilities include water, sugar water, apple water, lemonade, infusions of slippery elm or sassafrass pith, or solutions of gum
arabic, tapioca, or sage, to name only a few.

Protectives

Protectives are substances applied to a diseased part to protect it from contact with air or irritative substances generally. The function may be likened to nature's use of the scab to promote healing. Olive oil, lard, and wax may be applied directly for this purpose. Colloidon also has this function, in addition to serving as an adhesive to attach skin edges or dressings.

Pannier Medications of this class:

#45 Collodium
#25 Oleum Olivae
#25 Oleum Olivae

Antacids

Antacids are substances which correct acidity in whatever part of the body they encounter it, either through neutralization or by physical absorption. The most common use is correction of dyspepsia by correcting excess acidity of the stomach. They also serve for treatment of poisoning with acids (sulfuric, nitric, muriatic). They may also be helpful in sick headache (often due to gastric upset, with sympathy caused headache) and fever associated with a sour smell of the breath and sweat betraying the acid excess in the system. They are helpful for uric acid kidney and bladder stones.

Representatives include Carbonates of Potassa and Soda, Bicarbonates of Potassa and Soda, Liquor Ammoniae, Spirit of Ammoniae, lime water, Carbonate of Lime, and chalk.

Pannier Medications of this class:
#36 Potassae Bicarbonas
#19 Liquor Ammoniae

Medications in the Pannier

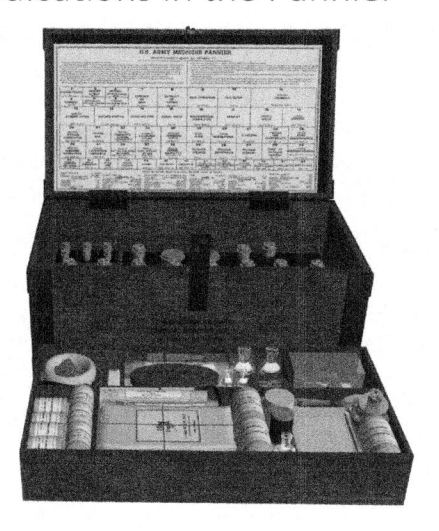

The medications supplied to (Federal) regimental surgeons packaged in the Medical Pannier represented what was felt to be the essential medications for treatment of the common diseases they were likely to encounter. For permanent hospitals and larger field hospitals additional medications could be supplied as per the official supply tables.

This section begins with a list, followed by each of the medications in the Pannier in detail, including their composition and use.

For each, an initial period references summarizes the use of the medication. Following this, set off in italics, is a modern perspective on that medication and its use, toxicity, and effectiveness, or lack thereof.

Finally, an extensive, detailed presentation of the medication drawn from period pharmacology text is available for further reference.

Bruce A. Evans, M.D.
ITEM NAMES

Pannier Medications

Pannier # and Formal Names with Common Names

#1 **Capisci Pulvis**
Chili Powder

#2 **Argenti Nitras**
Silver Nitrate Salt

#3 **Argenti Nitras Fusus**
Fused Silver Nitrate Crystals

#4 **Iodinium**
Iodine

#5 **Antimonii et Potassæ Tartras**
Tarter Emetic

#6 **Hydrargyri Chloridium Mite**
Calomel

#7 **Extract of Beef**

#8 **Extract of Coffee**

#9 **Milk, Condensed**

#10 **Tea, Black**

#11 **Spiritus Frumenti**
Whiskey

#12 **Spiritus Ætheris Nitrici**
Sweet Spirit of Nitre

#13 **Alcohol Fortius**
Strong Alcohol

#14 **Cough Mixture**

#15 **Sugar, White**

#16 **Chloroformum Purificatum**
Pure Chloroform

#17 **Liniment**

#18 **Syrupus Scillæ**
Syrup of Squill

#19 **Liquor Ammoniæ**
Ammonia Water

#20 **Spiritus Ætheris Compositus**
Compound Spirits of Sulphuric Ether
(Hoffman's Anodyne Liquor)

#21 **Tinctura Opii**
Tincture of Opium (Laudanum)

#22 **Tinctura Cinchonas Fluidum**
Tincture of Cinchona Bark

#23 **Extract Valerianæ Fluidum**
Extract of Valerian

#24 **Extract Zingiberis Fluidum**
Extract of Ginger Root

#25 **Oleum Olivæ**
Olive Oil

#26 **Oleum Terebinthinæ**
Oil of Turpentine

#27 **Glycerina**
Glycerin

#28 **Tinctura Opii Camphorata**
Camphorated Tincture of Opium (Paregoric)

#29 **Liquor Ferri Perisulphatus**
Ferric Persulphate Solution

#30 **Spiritus Ammoniæ Aromaticus**
Aromatic Spirits of Ammonia

#31 **Pilulæ Catharticæ Compositæ**
Compound Cathartic Pills

#32 **Pills of Colycin. Comp. and Ipecac**
Pills of Colocynth Compound Extract and Ipecac

#33 **Pills of Pulv. Ipecac et Opii**
Pills of Powdered Ipecac and Opium

#34 **Pilulæ Quiniæ Sulphatus**
Quinine Sulphate Pills

#35 **Potassæ Chloras**
Potassium Chlorate

#36 **Potassæ Bicarbonas**
Potassium Bicarbonate

#37 **Potassii Iodidum**
Iodide of Potassium

#38 **Sodæ et Potassæ Tartras**
Tartrate of Potassium and Soda (Rochelle Salt)

#39 **Liquor Morphiæ Sulphas**
Morphine Sulphate Solution

#40 **Pills of Camphor and Opium**
Pills of Camphorated Opium

#41 **Pilulæ Hydrargyri**
Mercury Pills (Blue Mass)

#42 **Pilulæ Opii**
Opium Pills

#43 **Acidum Tannicum**
Tannic Acid

#44 **Alumen**
Alum

#45 **Collodium**
Etheral Solution of Gun Cotton

#46 **Creasotum**
Creosote

#47 **Extractum Aconti Radicis Fluidum**
Fluid Extract of Aconite Root

#48 Extractum Colchici Seminis Fluidum
Fluid Extract of Colchicum Seed

#49 **Extractum Ipecacuanhæ Fluidum**
Fluid Extract of Ipecac

#50 **Tinctura Ferri Chloridi**
Ferric Chloride (Tincture of Muriate of Iron)

#51 **Plumbi Acetas**
Lead Acetate (Sugar of Lead)

#52 **Zinci Sulphas**
Zinc Sulphate (White Vitriol)

Ceratum Adipis
Simple Salve

Unguentum Hydragyri
Mercury Ointment

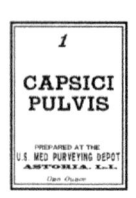

Capsici Pulvis (Chili powder) -
Yellowish to reddish brown powder; hot and fiery taste

This medication is used mainly in poultices and other skin applications for counter-stimulation, to reduce inflammation at a near or remote site, as in fever with delirium or coma and chronic rheumatism. The principle is that the capacity of the system to support inflammation is of a fixed degree, and if irritation is caused at the skin at a nearby or even remote site, the drawing of blood and congestion into that area will reduce the inflammation at the diseased area. Application of this substance causes local heat and redness, or with sufficient application, blistering. It is rarely used internally in bread pills as a stimulant to the stomach in torpid digestion

Modern Perspective:
This irritative substance was used to provoke an inflammatory reaction on the skin when applied in various ways and mixed with various adherent substance. In producing such a reaction it is certainly effective.
The presumed benefits of that reaction, in reducing pathologic inflammation in a contiguous area ("counter-irritation") or a distant site ("revulsion") , postulated from the theory that the patient's "system" could only sustain a fixed amount of inflammation and vascular excitement, are with modern knowledge, illusory.

Period Reference:

The Elements of Materia Medica and Therapeutics
Jonathan Pereira, M.D. (Blanchard and Lee,
Philadelphia, 1852) on the uses and administration of **Capsici Pulvis:**

Capsicum is more employed as a *condiment* than as a medicine. It is added to various articles of food, either to improve their flavour, or, if difficult of digestion, to promote their assimilation, and. to prevent flatulence. The inhabitants of tropical climates employ it to stimulate the digestive organs, and thereby to counteract the relaxing and enervating influence of external heat.

As a *medicine,* it is principally valuable as a local stimulant to the mouth, throat and stomach. Its constitutional not being in proportion to its topical effects, it is of little value as a general or diffusible stimulant. Administered internally, capsicum has long been esteemed in cases of *cynanche maligna.* It was used, in 1786, with great success by Mr. Stephens and by Mr. Collins. It promoted the separation of the sloughs, and soon improved the constitutional symptoms. Mr. Headby also employed it both internally and, by way of gargle. Its use has been extended to *scarlatina anginosa.* As a gargle, in relaxed conditions of the throat, its efficacy is undoubted. The powder or tincture may be applied, by means of a camel-hair pencil, to a relaxed uvula. It is a very useful gastric stimulant in enfeebled, languid, and torpid conditions of the stomach. Thus, in the dyspepsia of drunkards, as well as of gouty subjects, it has been found useful. In various diseases attended with diminished susceptibility of stomach, capsicum is an exceedingly useful adjunct to other powerful remedies, the operation of which it promotes by raising the dormant sensibility of this viscus; as in cholera, intermittents, low forms of fever, dropsies, &c. Dr. Wright speaks in high terms of it as a remedy for obviating the black vomit — a symptom of the fever of tropical climates, at one time considered fatal. A capsicum cataplasm may be used with advantage to occasion rubefaction in any cases in which a rubefacient counter-irritant is indicated; as in the coma and delirium of fever, in chronic rheumatism, &c.; unless kept on for a long period it does not vesicate.

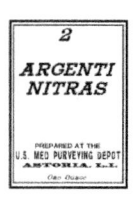

Argenti Nitras (silver nitrate, white salt) -
White powder

This is used as an escharotic in solution for external use, to cause scarring and subsequent healing of chronic ulcers and sores, including mercury induced mouth lesions. It is useful for changing the character of the surface - changing a weeping surface to a dry scar - to promote healing in foul or sloughing sores, especially when there is only a surface tendency to gangrene with healthy deep tissues, as this application has a surface action only.

Modern Perspective:

Silver nitrate is a powerful oxidizing agent and is still used to cauterized skin and mucous membrane lesions. In addition, silver has an antibacterial effect, and any metallic silver formed from the ionic form by the oxidation-reduction reaction responsible for the caustic effect may have contributed to (a then unappreciated) protective effect against subsequent bacterial infection of the wound.

Some modern bandages are impregnated with metallic silver due to the antibacterial effect.

Period Reference:

Bruce A. Evans, M.D.

The Elements of Materia Medica and Therapeutics – Jonathan Pereira, M.D. (Blanchard and Lee, Philadelphia, 1852) on the uses and administration of:

Silver Nitrate

Uses.– Nitrate of silver has been employed *internally* in a very few cases only; and of these the principal and most important are epilepsy, chorea, and angina pectoris. Its liability to discolour the skin is a great drawback to its use; indeed, I conceive that a medical man is not justified in risking the production of this effect without previously informing his patient of the possible result. Dr. Osborne ascribes its good effects to its allaying irritation of the gastric membrane. But in a larger number of instances the asserted. existence of this irritation is a mere as assumption, perfectly devoid of proof.

In *epilepsy,* it has occasionally, perhaps more frequently than any other remedy, proved successful. Drs. Sims, Baillie, R. Harrison, Roget, and. J. Johnson have all borne testimony to its beneficial effects. Its *methodus medendi* is imperfectly understood. This, indeed, is to be expected, when it is considered that the pathology and causes of epilepsy are so little known; and that, as Dr. Sims has justly observed, everything concerning this disease is involved in the greatest doubt and obscurity, if we except the descriptions of a single fit, and that it returns at uncertain intervals. In this state of ignorance, and with the already-mentioned facts before us, as to the curative powers of this salt, the observation of Georget, that he has great difficulty in conceiving how the blindest empiricism should have led any one to attempt the cure of a diseased brain by cauterizing the stomach, is, I conceive, most absurd and unwarranted. The cases which have been relieved by it are probably those termed by Br. M. Hall eccentric. In the few instances in which I have seen this remedy tried, it has proved unsuccessful; but it was not continued long, on account of the apprehended discoloration of the skin.

In *chorea,* it has been successfully employed by Dr. Powell, Dr. Uwins, Dr. Crampton, Lombard, and others. In *angina pectoris,* it has been administered in the intervals of the paroxysms with occasional success by Dr. Cappe and Dr. Copland.

In *chronic affections of the stomach* (especially morbid sensibility of the gastric and intestinal nerves), it has been favourably spoken of by Autenrieth, Dr. James Johnson, and Rueff. It has been employed to allay chronic vomiting connected with disordered innervation, as well as with disease of the stomach (scirrhus and cancer), and to relieve gastrodynia. The foregoing are the most important of the diseases against which nitrate of silver has been administered internally.

As an *external agent,* its uses are far more valuable, while they are free from the inconvenience of permanently staining the skin. It is employed sometimes as a *caustic,* and. as such it has some advantages over potassa fusa and the liquid corrosives. Thus, it does not liquefy by its application, and hence its action is confined to the parts with which it is placed in contact. It is used to remove and repress spongy granulations in wounds aud ulcers, and to destroy warts, whether venereal or otherwise. It is applied to chancres on their first appearance, with the view of decomposing the syphilitic poison, and thereby of stopping its absorption, and preventing bubo or secondary symptoms. This practice has the sanction of Mr. Hunter. I have several times seen it fail, perhaps because it was not adopted sufficiently early. The nitrate should be scraped to a point, and applied to every part of the

ulcer. This mode of treating chancres has been recently brought forward *by* Ratier, as if it were new, and as forming part of Bretonneau's *ectrotic (ectrotica,* from the greek for *I abort)* method of treating diseases!

The application of nitrate of silver to *punctured wounds* is often attended with most beneficial effect, as Mr. Higginbottom has fully proved. It prevents or subdues inflammatory action in a very surprising manner. It is equally adapted for poisoned as for simple wounds. To promote the healing of *ulcers,* it is a most valuable remedy. In large indolent ulcers, particularly those of a fistulous or callous kind, it acts as a most efficient stimulant. To small ulcers it may be applied so as to cause an eschar, and when at length this peels off, the sore is found to be healed. Mr. Higginbottom asserts that "in every instance in which the eschar remains adherent from the first application, the wound or ulcer over which it is formed invariably heals. Dry lint will, in general, be found the best dressing for sores touched with the nitrate.

Nitrate of silver was proposed. by Mr. Higginbottom as a topical remedy for external inflammation. It may be applied with great advantage to subdue the inflammatory action of erythema, of paronychia or whitlow, and of inflamed absorbents. In some cases, it is merely necessary to blacken the cuticle; in others, Mr. Higginbottom recommends it to be used so as to induce vesication. In erysipelas, nitrate of silver is used. by many surgeons as a cautery both to the inflamed and the surrounding healthy parts. Mr. Higginbottom uses in erysipelas a solution composed of Argenti Nitr. four scruples; Acidi Nitrici six drops; Distilled Water four scruples. But I have so often seen the disease continue its course as if nothing had been done, that I have lost confidence in its efficacy. I have found tincture of iodine much preferable.

Bretonneau and Serres recommend the *cauterization of variolous pustules by* nitrate of silver, in order to cut short their progress. It is principally useful as a means of preventing pitting, and should be employed on the first or second. day of the eruption. The solid caustic is to be applied to each pustule after the apices have been removed. This ectrotic method has also been employed in the treatment of *shingles* (herpes zoster): in one case the disease was cured in a few hours. Some good rules for its application have been laid down by Rayer.

In some diseases of the eye, nitrate of silver is a most valuable remedial agent. It is used in the solid state in solution and in ointment: the solution may be used as a wash or injection, or applied by a camel's hair pencil. In deep ulcers of the cornea, a cone of the solid nitrate should be applied – in superficial ones, a solution (of from four to ten grains of the salt to an ounce of distilled water) may be employed. There is one drawback to the use of this substance in ulcers of the cornea, as well as other affections of the eye: viz. the danger of producing dark specks in the cornea, or of staining the conjunctiva, but this occurrence is rare. Velpeau has employed it in many hundred cases without ever observing such an effect. In both acute and chronic ophthalmia, Mr. Guthrie employs this salt in the form of ointment. Of this, he directs a portion (varying in size from a large pin's head to that of a garden pea) to be introduced. between the lids by the finger or a camel's hair pencil. It causes more or less pain, which sometimes lasts only half an hour, at others till next day. Warm anodyne fomentations are to be used, and. the application of the ointment repeated every third day. In acute cases, two or three applications will arrest the disease. With this treatment, bloodletting, and the use of

calomel and opium, are preceded or conjoined. While many surgeons hesitate to use nitrate of silver in the first stage of acute purulent ophthalmia, all are agreed. as to its value in the second stage of the disease, as well as in chronic ophthalmia. Besides the diseases of the eye already mentioned, there are many others in which the oculist finds this salt of the greatest service as a caustic, astringent, or stimulant.

In *inflammatory affections and ulcerations of the mucous membrane of the mouth and fauces,* nitrate of silver is sometimes a most valuable application. When the fibrinous exudation of croup commences on the surface of the tonsil and. arches of the palate, its further progress may be stopped, according to Mr. Mackenzie, by the application of a solution composed of a scruple of nitrate of silver and. an ounce of distilled water. The solid nitrate has been introduced through an aperture in the trachea, and. applied to ulcers on the inner surface of the larynx, in a case of phthisis laryngea, with apparent benefit.

In some forms of *leucorrhoea,* the application of nitrate of silver, either in the solid. state or in solution, is attended with beneficial effects. This practice was first recommended by Dr. Jewel. It is, I believe, most successful in cases dependent on local irritation or subacute inflammation, and not arising from constitutional debility. The solution may be applied by a piece of lint or sponge, or may be injected by means of a syringe with a curved pipe. Its strength must vary according to circumstances. Dr. Jewel generally employed three grains of the nitrate to an ounce of water; but in the Lock Hospital, solutions are sometimes used containing half a drachm, or even two scruples, to the ounce. In some cases the solid nitrate has been applied to the cervix uteri and vagina by means of a silver tube. In *gonorrhoea, of the female,* a solution of the nitrate of silver, or even this caustic in the solid state, has been used with the best effects. It was first employed by Dr. Jewel; but subsequently, and on a much more extended scale, by Dr. Hannay and without any injurious consequences. In many cases the discharge ceased, never to return, in twenty-four hours. The fear of ill effects has prevented the general adoption of this practice. In *gonorrhoea of the male,* the introduction of a bougie, smeared. with an ointment of nitrate of silver, is occasionally a most effectual cure; but the practice is dangerous. In one case I saw acute and nearly fatal urethritis brought on by its employment. The patient was a dresser at one of the Lond.on hospitals, and had practiced this mode of treatment in many instances on the hospital patients with the happiest results. An aqueous solution of the salt has been successfully used in chronic gonorrhea.

In *fissured or excoriated nipples,* the application of the solid. nitrate of silver is of great service. It should be insinuated into all the chaps or cracks, and the nipple afterwards washed with tepid milk and. water.

The application of solid nitrate of silver is a most effectual remedy for the different forms of *porrigo* which affect the heads of children. The caustic should be well rubbed into the parts. l have never known the practice to fail, or to cause the loss of hair. Where the greater portion of the scalp is involved, the different spots should be cauterized. successively at intervals of some days; for, as already mentioned, I have seen fever and delirium produced in a child from the too excessive use of this remedy. In *psoriasis,* the same medicine was found by Dr. Graves most effectual. An aqueous solution of the nitrate is also valuable as an astringent wash in other skin diseases, as *impetigo.* The solid nitrate is sometimes employed. to stop the progress of irritative or erysipelatous inflammation, by applying it in a circular form around, and at a little distance from, the inflamed portion; but I have frequently observed the inflammation extend beyond the cauterized part. Mr. Higginbottom reports favourably of the effects of applying the nitrate to *burns* and *scalds;* and his observations have been confirmed by those of Mr. Cox.

In *strictures of the urethra and oesophagus,* bougies armed with lunar caustic on their points *(the caustic* or *armed bougie)* are occasionally employed with great advantage, at least in urethral stricture. When the common bougie *(cereolus simplex)* is formed, the point of it should be heated with a conical piercer, and the caustic introduced while the composition is quite soft. The point of the bougie should then be rubbed quite smooth on a piece of polished. marble till no inequality in the size of it appear. Notwithstanding that the application of nitrate of silver to stricture of the urethra has been advocated by Mr. Hunter, Sir K. Home, *Mr.* Wilson, Dr. Andrews, and others, it is now but little employed.; yet of its efficacy and safety in many obstinate cases, where the simple bougie fails, I am assured by repeated observation. It is commonly supposed. that it acts by burning or destroying the stricture: such is not the fact. It induces some change in the vital actions of the part, which is followed. by a relaxation of the narrowed portion of the canal, but which change is as difficult to explain as the subduction of the internal inflammatory action by the application of this salt. Of the use of the caustic bougie in stricture of the oesophagus I have no experience.

Administration.– Nitrate of silver may be exhibited in doses of one-sixth of a grain, gradually increased to three or four grains, three times a day. As before mentioned, Dr. Powell has increased the dose to fifteen grains. The usual mode of administering it is in the form of pills made of bread-crumb; but the chloride. of sodium which it contains renders it objectionable: some mild vegetable powder with mucilage is preferable. Common salt or salted food should not be taken either immediately before or after swallowing these pills. Dr. Johnson asserts "that there is no instance on record where the complexion has been affected by the medicine when restricted to three months' administration." It is advisable, however, not to continue the use of it beyond a month or six weeks at a time.

For external use, an aqueous solution is employed of strengths varying from a quarter of a grain to two scruples, in an ounce of distilled water.

Antidote.– The antidote for nitrate of silver is common salt *(chloride of sodium)*. When this comes in contact with lunar caustic, nitrate of soda and chloride of silver are produced: the latter compound is, according to the experiments of Orna, innocuous. The contents of the stomach should be removed, and. the inflammatory symptoms combated by demulcents, bloodletting, and the usual antiphlogistic means.

When the local use of nitrate of silver causes excessive pain, relief may be gained by washing the parts with a solution of common salt. Pieces of caustic have been left in the vagina and urethra without unpleasant consequences resulting. Injections of a solution of common salt are the best means of preventing bad effects.

To diminish the slate-coloured tint of the skin arising from nitrate of silver, acids or the super-salts offer the most probable means of success. The external and internal use of dilute nitric acid, or the internal employment of bitartrate of potash, may be tried: the discoloration is said. to have yielded to a steady course of the last-mentioned substance.

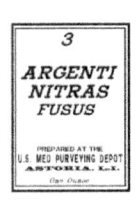

Argenti Nitras Fusus (fused silver nitrate)

Similar to Argenti Nitras except supplied as large crystals rather than powder. For external use; applied to skin lesions while gripped in a caustic holder (component of the pocket case).

Modern Perspective:

Silver nitrate is a powerful oxidizing agent and is still used to cauterized skin and mucous membrane lesions. In addition, silver has an antibacterial effect, and any metallic silver formed from the ionic form by the oxidation-reduction reaction responsible for the caustic effect may have contributed to (a then unappreciated) protective effect against subsequent bacterial infection of the wound.

Some modern bandages are impregnated with metallic silver due to the antibacterial effect.

This form was created by fusing the salt into a larger mass, for use (in a "caustic holder") to touch and cauterize lesions.

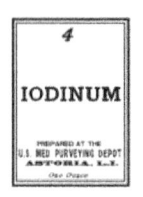

```
    4
IODINUM
PREPARED AT THE
U.S. MED PURVEYING DEPOT
  ASTORIA, L.I.
     One Ounce
```

Iodinium (Iodine) -
Bluish-black crystal with metallic luster, odor resembling chlorine

Iodinium is used as a corrosive and irritant in local application for scrofula, ulcer, erysipelas, and chilblains. Placed out in open pans to provide disinfectant for hospital wards. For external use, especially in erysipelas, the tincture (prepared as a solution of iodine in alcohol) is sometimes used as a paint.

Modern Perspective:

This was mainly used externally, utilizing its corrosive effect against various types of skin lesions.

It was also felt to have disinfectant properties, although the understanding of that term was different than the current implication of preventing bacterial infection. Disinfectants were applied to inflamed wounds to retard "mortification" - the progression to tissue death associated with the sloughing off of dead tissue and "fetid" smells. The concept of applying disinfectants prior to inflammatory change - what we would recognize as infection - to prevent that occurance was unknown until Lister publicized the use of such a substance - phenolic or carbolic acid - for just that purpose, and revolutionized the practice of surgery.

The use of this substance in pans throughout the hospitals begins, however, to hint at this kind of preventative use. Unfortunately, such use had more effect at covering up the smells of various infections than preventing their occurrence or spread.

Period Reference:

M.D. (Blanchard and Lee, Philadelphia, 1852) on the uses and administration of:
Iodine

Uses.– As a remedial agent iodine is principally valuable for its resolvent influence in chronic visceral and glandular enlargements, indurations, thickening of membranes (as of the periosteum), and in tumours. In comparing its therapeutical power with that of mercury, we observe in the first place that it is not adapted for febrile and acute inflammatory complaints, in several of which mercury proves a most valuable agent. Indeed, the existence of inflammatory fever is a contraindication for the employment of iodine. Secondly, iodine is especially adapted for scrofulous, mercury for syphilitic, maladies; and it is well known that in the former class of diseases mercurials are for the most part injurious. Thirdly, the influence of iodine over the secreting organs is much less constant and powerful than that of mercury: so that, in retention or suppression of the secretions, mercury is for the most part greatly superior to iodine. Fourthly, iodine evinces a specific influence over the diseases of certain organs (e. g. the thyroid body), which mercury does not.– These are some only of the peculiarities which distinguish the therapeutical action of iodine from that of mercury.

In *bronchocele–* Of all the remedies yet proposed for bronchocele, this has been by far the most successful. Indeed, judging only from the numerous cases cured by it, and which have been published, we should almost infer it to be a sovereign remedy. However, of those who have written on the use of iodine in this complaint, some only have published a numerical list of their successful and unsuccessful cases. Bayle has given a summary of those published by Coster, Irmenger, Baup, and Manson, from which it appears that, of 364 cases treated by iodine, 274 were cured. Dr. Copland observes that, of several cases of the disease which have come before him since the introduction of this remedy into practice, "there has not been one which has not either been cured or remarkably relieved by it." I much regret, however, that my own experience does not accord with this statement. I have repeatedly seen iodine, given in conjunction with iodide of potassium, and used both externally and internally, fail in curing bronchocele; and I know others whose experience has been similar. Dr. Bardsley cured only nine, and relieved six, out of thirty cases, with iodide of potassium. To what circumstances, then, ought we to attribute this variable result? Dr. Copland thinks that, where it fails, it has been given in "too large and irritating doses, or in an improper form; and, without due attention having been paid to certain morbid and constitutional relations of the disease during the treatment."

But, in two or three of the instances before mentioned, I believe the failure did not arise from any of the circumstances alluded to by Dr. Copland, and I am disposed to refer it to some peculiar condition of the tumour, or of the constitution. When we consider that the terms *bronchocele, goitre,* and *Derbyshire neck,* are applied to very different conditions of the thyroid gland, and that the causes which produce them are involved in great obscurity, and may, therefore, be, and indeed probably are, as diversified as the conditions they give rise to, we can easily imagine that, while iodine is serviceable in some, it may be useless, or even injurious, in others. Sometimes the bronchocele consists in hypertrophy of the substance of the thyroid gland – that is, this organ is enlarged, but has a healthy structure. In others, the tumefaction of the gland takes place suddenly, and may even disappear as suddenly; from which it has been inferred that the enlargement depends on an accumulation of blood in the vessels, and an elusion of serum into its tissue. Coindet mentions a goitre which was developed excessively during the first pregnancy of a young female: twelve hours after her accouchement it had entirely disappeared. The same author also relates the circumstance of a regiment composed of young recruits, who were almost every man attacked with considerable enlargement of the thyroid gland, shortly after their arrival at Geneva, where they all drank water out of the same pump. On their quarters being changed the gland soon regained its natural size in every instance. A third class of bronchoceles consists of an enlargement of the thyroid gland from the development of certain fluid or solid substances in its interior, and which may be contained in cells, or be infiltrated through its substance. These accidental productions may be serous, honey-like, gelatinous, fibrous, cartilaginous, or osseous. Lastly, at times the enlarged gland has acquired a scirrhous condition. Now it is impossible that all these different conditions can be cured with equal facility by iodine; those having solid deposits are, of course, most difficult to get rid of. Kolley, who was himself cured of a large goitre of ten years' standing, says that, for the iodine to be useful, the bronchocele should not be of too long standing, nor painful to the touch; the swelling confined to the thyroid gland, and not of a scirrhous or carcinomatous nature, nor containing any stony or other analogous concretions; and that the general health be not disordered by any febrile or inflammatory symptoms, or any gastric, hepatic, or intestinal irritation. If the swelling be tender to the touch, and have other marks of inflammation, let the usual local antiphlogistic measures precede the employment of iodine. When this agent is employed, we may administer it both externally and internally. The most effectual method of employing iodine externally is that called. *endermic,* already described; namely, to apply an ioduretted ointment (usually containing iodide of potassium) to the cutis vera, the epidermis being previously removed by a blister. But the *epidermic* or *iatroleptic* method is more usually followed – that is, the ioduretted ointment is rubbed into the affected part, without the epidermis being previously removed, or the undiluted tincture is repeatedly applied to the part by a camel's- hair pencil, while iodine is at the same time administered internally. With respect to the internal use of this substance, some think that the success depends on the use of small doses largely diluted; while others consider that as large a quantity of the remedy should be administered as the stomach and general system can bear.

b. Scrofula is another disease for which iodine has been extensively used. " Dr. Coindet was, I believe, the first to direct public attention to this remedy in the disease in question. Subsequently,

Baup, Gimelle, Kolley, Sablairoles, Bena- ben, Callaway, and others, published cases illustrative of its beneficial effects. Dr. Manson deserves the credit of having first tried it on an extensive scale. He treated upwards of eighty cases of scrofula and scrofulous ophthalmia by the internal exhibition of iodine, sometimes combined with its external employment; and in a large proportion of cases, where the use of the medicine was persevered in, the disease was either cured or ameliorated, the general health being also improved. Three memoirs on the effects of iodine in scrofula have been subsequently published by Lugol, physician to the Hopital St.Louis, serving to confirm the opinions already entertained of its efficacy. From the first memoir it appears that in seventeen months – namely, from August 1827, to December 1828 – 109 scrofulous patients were treated by iodine only; and. that of these 86 were completely cured, and 30 relieved; in 4 cases the treatment was ineffectual, and 39 cases were under treatment at the time of the report made by Serres, Magendie, and Dumeril, to the Academie Royale des Sciences. In his illustrative cases we find glandular swellings, scrofulous ophthalmia, abscesses, ulcers, and diseases of the bones, were beneficially treated by it. Lugol employs iodine internally and externally: for internal administration, he prefers iodine dissolved in water by means of iodide of potassium, given either in the form of *drops,* or largely diluted, under the form of what he calls *ioduretted mineral water,* hereafter to be described. His external treatment is of two kinds; one for the purpose of obtaining local effects only, the other for procuring constitutional or general effects. His local external treatment consists in employing ointments or solutions of iodine: the *ointments* are made either with iodine and iodide of potassium, or with the protiodide of mercury; the *solutions* are of iodine and iodide of potassium in water; and according to their strength are denominated caustic, rubefacient, or stimulant: the rubefacient solu- tion is employed in making cataplasms and local baths. His external general treatment consists in the employment of *ioderetted baths.* In the treatment of cutaneous scrofula, I have seen the most beneficial results from the application of the tincture of iodine by means of a camel's-hair pencil. It dries up the discharge and. promotes cicatrization. The successful results obtained by Lugol in the treatment of this disease cannot, I think, in many instances, be referred to iodine solely. Many of the patients were kept several months (some as much as a year) under treatment in the hospital, where every attention was paid to the improvement of their general health by warm clothing, good diet, the use of vapour and sulphur-baths, &c.; means which of them- selves are sufficient to ameliorate, if not cure, many of the scrofulous conditions before alluded to. Whether it be to the absence of these supplementary means of diet and regimen, or to some other cause, I know not, but most practitioners will, I think, admit that they cannot obtain, by the use of iodine, the same successful results which Lugol is said to have met with, though in a large number of cases this agent has been found a most useful remedy.

c. Iodine has been eminently successful when employed as a resolvent *in chronic diseases of various organs, especially those accompanied with induration and enlargement. By* some inexplicable influence, it sometimes not only puts a stop to the further progress of disease, but apparently restores the part to its normal state. It is usually given with the view of exciting the action of the absorbents, but its influence is not limited to this set of vessels: it exercises a controlling and modifying influence over the bloodvessels of the affected part, and is in the true sense of the word an *alterative* (see *ante,* pp. 214 – 215). In chronic inflammation, induration, and enlargement of the *liver,* after antiphlogistic measures have been adopted, the two most important and probable means of relief are iodine and mercury, which may be used either separately or conjointly. If the disease admit of a cure, these are the agents most likely to effect it. Iodine, indeed, has been supposed to possess some specific power of influencing the liver, not only from its efficacy in alleviating or curing certain diseases of this organ but also from the effects of an over-dose. In one case, pain and induration of the liver were brought on; and in another, which terminated fatally, this organ was found to be enlarged, and of a pale rose colour. Several cases of enlarged *spleens* relieved, or cured, by iodine have been published. In chronic diseases of the *uterus,* accompanied with induration and enlargement, iodine has been most successfully employed. In 1828, a remarkable instance was published. by Dr. Thetford. The uterus was of osseous hardness, and of so considerable a size as nearly to fill the whole of the pelvis: yet in six weeks the disease had given way to the use of iodine, and the catamenia was restored. In the *Guy's Hospital Reports,* No. I. 1836, is an account, by Dr. Ashwell, of seven case of "hard tumours" of the uterus successfully treated by the use of iodine, in conjunction with occasional depletion, and regulated and mild. diet. Besides the internal use of iodine, this substance was employed, in the form of ointment (composecd of iodine gr. xv, iodide potassium 2 scruples, spermaceti oint. one and one-half fluid ounce), of which a portion (about the size of a nutmeg) was introduced into the vagina, and rubbed into the affected cervix for ten or twelve minutes every night. It may be applied by the finger, or by a camel's-hair pencil, or sponge mounted on a slender piece of cane. The average time in which resolution of the induration is accomplished varies, according to Dr. Ashwell, from eight to sixteen weeks. "In hard tumours of the walls or cavity of the uterus, resolution, or disappearance, is scarcely to be expected;" but "hard tumours of the cervix, and indurated puckerings of the edges of the os (conditions which most frequently terminate in ulceration) may be melted down and cured by the iodine." In *ovarian* tumours, iodine has been found serviceable. In the *chronic mammary tumour,* described by Sir A.. Cooper, I have seen it give great relief – alleviating pain, and keeping the disease in check. In *indurated enlargements of the paro- tid, prostate, and lymphatic glands,* several successful cases of its use have been. published.

d. As an *emmenagogue,* iodine has been recommended by Coindet, Brera; Sablairoles, Magendie, and others. The last-mentioned writer tells us that, on one occasion, he gave it to a young lady, whose propriety of conduct he had no reason to doubt, and that she miscarried after using it for three weeks. I have known, it given for a bronchocele during pregnancy without having the least obvious influence over the uterus.

e. In *gonorrhoea* and *leucorrhoea,* it has been employed with success after the inflammatory symptoms have subsided.

f. inhalation of *iodine vapour* has been used in phthisis and chronic bronchitis. In the first of these diseases it has been recommended by Berton, Sir James Mur- ray, and Sir Charles Scudamore. I have repeatedly tried it in this as well as in other chronic pulmonary complaints, but never with the least benefit. The apparatus for inhaling it is the same as that used for the inhalation of chlorine (see *ante,* p. 382). The liquid employed is a solution of ioduretted iodide of potassium, to which, Sir C. Scudamore adds the tincture of conium.

g. Chronic diseases of the nervous system, such as paralysis and chorea, have been successfully treated by iodine by Dr. Manson.

h. In some forms of *the venereal disease,* iodine has been found a most serviceable remedy. Thus Richond (quoted by Bayle) employed. it, after the usual antiphlogistic measures, to remove buboes. De Salle cured chronic venereal affections of the testicles with it. Mr. Mayo has pointed out its efficacy in certain disorders which are the consequences of syphilis, such as emaciation of the frame, with ulcers of the skin; ulcerated throat; and inflammation of the bones, or periosteum – occurring in patients to whom mercury has been given.

i. In checking or controlling the ulcerative process, iodine is, according to Mr. Key, one of the most powerful remedies we possess. " The most active phagedenic ulcers, that threaten the destruction of parts, are often found to yield in a surprising manner to the influence of this medicine, and to put on a healthy granulating appearance."

j. Resides the diseases already mentioned, there are many others in which iodine has been used with considerable advantage: for example – *chronic skin diseases,* as lepra, psoriasis, &c.' (I have seen it aggravate psoriasis); – *dropsies, in old non- united fractures,* to promote the deposition of ossific matter," and *in chronic rheumatism;* but, in the latter disease, iodide of potassium is more frequently employed. *As an antidote in poisoning by strychnia, brucita,* and *veratria,* iodine has been recommended by M. Ronnd, because the compound formed by the union of these alkalies with iodine is less active than the alkalies themselves: as an *injection for the cure of hydrocele,* Velpeau has employed a mixture of the tincture of iodine with water, in the proportion of from one to two drachms of the tincture to an ounce of water: of this mixture from one to four ounces are to be injected and imme- diately withdrawn; lastly, to check *mercurial salivation* iodine has been successfully used.

    h. As a *topical remedy* iodine is exceedingly valuable in several classes of diseases. Dr. Davies, of Hertford, has drawn the attention of the profession to its employment in this way, and pointed out the great benefit attending it. In most cases the tincture is the preparation employed. The part affected is painted with this liquid by means of a camel's-hair pencil. In some few cases only, where the skin is very delicate, will it be necessary to dilute the preparation. When it is required to remove the stain which its use gives rise to, a poultice or gruel should be applied. In *lupus* it proves highly beneficial. My attention was first drawn to its efficacy in this disease by my colleague Mr. Luke. Under its employment the process of ulceration is generally stopped, and cicatrization takes place. The tincture should be applied not only to the ulcerated portion, but to the parts around. In *eczema* it also is an excellent application. In *cutaneous scrofula,,* likewise, as I have already remarked. In several other cutaneous diseases, such as *lichen, prurigo, pityriasis, psoriasis, impetigo, porrigo, ecthyme,* and *scabies,* Dr. Kennedy has found its use beneficial. According to the testimony of Dr. Davies and an anonymous writer, it is a valuable application to *chilblains.* In the treatment of *diseases of the joints* it is used with great advantage. In *erysipelas* I have seen it highly benefcial. In *phlegmonous inflammation, sloughing of the cellular membrane, inflammation of the absorbents, gout, carbuncle, whitlow, lacerated, contused and punctured wounds,* and *burns* and *scalds,* it is most highly spoken of by Dr. Davies. In *acute rheumatism* and *gout* the application of iodine to the affected parts gives unquestionable relief. Either tincture of iodine or iodine paint (to be described. presently) should be applied to the affected. joints by means of a camel's-hair pencil, and repeated daily until the cuticle begins to peel off. According to my experience, no remedy gives so much relief as this: I have rarely found it fail. It deserves, however, especial notice, that the skin of different invalids is most unequally susceptible of its influence; in some few it excites so much pain that a second application of it is with difficulty permitted. In others, however, it produces scarcely any painful effects. In *diseases of the lungs and bronchial tubes* simulating phthisis, and also in incipient protracted phthisis, it may be applied to the outside of the thorax with great benefit. It is usually a much less painful application than emetic tartar or croton, oil, though, as I believe, equally effective. Its topical uses are, therefore, nearly as extensive as those of nitrate of silver. Moreover, it is used very much in the same classes of cases, and with the same views. **Administration**. – Iodine is rarely administered alone, but generally in con- junction with *iodide of potassium,* to the account of which substance I must refer for formulae for the combined exhibition of these substances. In the administration of iodine, care should be taken to avoid gastric irritation.

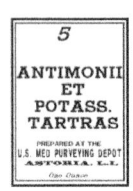

Antimonii et Potassæ Tartras (Tarter Emetic) - Transparent, colorless crystal becoming white and opaque with age
(Use has been documented since 1631)

The medicine is best given diluted in water. Small doses (one-twelfth to one-quarter grain every 2 to 3 hours) calm the pulse and respiration and increase secretions. With larger doses (up to ½ grain every hour or two), more profuse effect on the secretions and nausea will result. These changes benefit fever (especially when given with salt solutions) and other symptoms of inflammation, in doses too small to cause vomiting. This is the most efficient remedy existing for early stages of inflammation, especially with fever. If the skin is dry and hot, and benefit from increased sweating would be expected, the patient may be covered and given medicine to promote sweating (**Spiritus Ætheris Nitrici**); copious sweating will result. It is contraindicated, due to a direct irritative effect, on inflammation of the stomach and bowels. Wood states it should be used as an adjunct, not substitution, for depletion by bleeding or purging in treatment of the phlegmasiæ.

Modern Perspective:

There is no getting around the fact that Tartar Emetic does cause copious sweating and energetic vomiting. Unfortunately, we now know that inducing these effects has no benefit for the "inflammatory" diseases treated by the civil war surgeon, most of which were infectious in nature, and respond best, and sometimes only, to specific treatment of the responsible organism. On the other hand, it is an effective emetic - if not worth the toxicity - and remained in general medical use into the 20th century. This drug, along with the mercurials, long retained an almost mystical faith by practitioners that it somehow benefited a range of serious diseases.

The toxicity level of this drug is great. The minimun lethal dose (if not vomited up) is 2 grains; the emetic dose is one-half grain.

The toxicity is quite similar to arsenic poisoning. Drug induced inflammation of the stomach can lead to bleeding and possibly shock and death, from vascular collapse. Dizziness, muscle spasms, and delirium accompanied by headache may also occur. The drug also damages the kidney, the liver, and nerves.

Period Reference:

The Elements of Materia Medica and Therapeutics – Jonathan Pereira, M.D. (Blanchard and Lee, Philadelphia, 1852) on the uses and administration of:
Tartar Emetic

Uses – As an *emetic,* this salt is usually administered by the stomach, but it is sometimes used as an enema, and occasionally is injected into the' veins. When administered by the stomach, it is generally given in doses of one or two grains, frequently in combination with ten or fifteen grains of ipecacuanha. When our object is merely to evacuate the contents of the stomach, and with as little constitutional disorder as possible (as in cases of narcotic poisoning), other emetics (as the sulphates of zinc and copper) are to be preferred, since they occasion less nausea and depression of system, while they excite speedy vomiting. On the other hand, when we use vomiting as a means of making an impression on the system, and thereby of putting a sudden stop to the progress of a disease, emetic tartar is by far our best vomit. It is with this view that it is sometimes employed in the early stages of fever, especially when accompanied by gastric or bilious disorder. Emetic tartar is used as a vomit, with considerable success, in the early stage of inflammatory diseases; especially in croup, tonsillitis, swelled testicle, bubo, and ophthalmia. Here, also, the success of the remedy is in proportion to its early application. In croup it should be given to excite in the erst instance vomiting, and afterwards prolonged nausea. Under this plan of treatment, I have seen two or three slight cases completely recover without the use of any other remedial agent. Dr. Copland also bears testimony to the success of. the practice. In most cases it will be found advisable to precede the use of this medicine by bloodletting. Dr. Cheyne advises the employment of emetic tartar, in the second stage of croup, for the purpose of moderating vascular action, and of promoting' the separation of the adventitious membrane. Rut I am disposed to rely chiefly on calomel (given so as speedily to occasion ptyalism) and blood-letting. Dr. Cheyne recommends half a grain of emetic tartar to be dissolved in a tablespoonful of water, and given to a child, two or three years of age, every half hour till sickness and vomiting are produced; and, in two hours after the last act of vomiting, the same process is to be recommenced, and. so repeated while the strength will admit. Another disease which is relieved by the occasional use of emetics is *hooping-cough.* They should be administered at the commencement of the disease, every, or every other day. They diminish the violence and length of the fits of spasmodic coughing, and promote expectoration. Emetic tartar is particularly valuable in this disease, *in con*sequence of being tasteless, and, therefore, peculiarly adapted for exhibition to children. In derangements of the hepatic functions indicating the employment of emetics, this salt is usually preferred to other vomiting agents, on account of its supposed influence in promoting the secretion of bile.

    Clysters containing emetic tartar have been employed to occasion vomiting, but they are very uncertain in their operation. Rayer has frequently employed from six to twelve grains without producing either nausea or vomiting.
It has been repeatedly *injected into the veins* to excite vomiting. The usual dose is two or three grains dissolved in two ounces of water; but in some cases six grains have been employed. The effects are unequal: when vomiting does occur, it is not always immediate; frequently it

does not take place at all. In several cases of choking, from the lodgment of pieces of meat in the esophagus, this remedy has been applied with great success: vomiting was produced, and with it the expulsion of the meat. It has also been tried in epilepsy and trismus; but frequently with dangerous consequences. Meckel employed it to restore animation in asphyxia by drowning. It has also been used in tetanus.

As a *nauseant,* to reduce the force of the circulation and the muscular power, emetic tartar is frequently of considerable service. Thus, in dislocations of the larger joints (the hip and shoulder, for example), bloodletting, and nauseating doses of emetic tartar, are employed to diminish the resistance of the muscles opposing the reduction. Even in strangulated hernia it has been given.'

Emetic tartar, in large doses, is a most powerful and valuable remedy in the treatment of inflammation. On this subject I have already offered some remarks (see *ante,* pp. 228 and 224). As an emetic, nauseant, or diaphoretic, it has long been in use in peripneumonia; having been employed by Riverius in the 17th century, and subsequently by Stoll, Rrendel, Schroeder, and Richter, in Germany; by Pringle, Cullen, and Marryat, in England. But as a remedy for inflammation independent of its evacuant effects, we are indebted for it to Rasori, who first used it in the years 1799 and 1800, in an epidemic fever which raged at Genoa. Subsequently he exhibited it much more extensively, and in larger doses, in peripneumonia. This mode of treatment was tried and adopted in France, first by Laennec and in this country by Dr. Balfour. Its value as an antiphlogistic is now almost universally admitted. Practitioners, however, are not quite agreed as to the best method of using it. Rasori, Laennec, Reeamier, Rroussais, Bouillaud, Dr. Mackintosh, Drs. Graves and Stokes, Dr. Davies, and most practitioners of this country, employ bloodletting in peripneumonia, in conjunction with the use of emetic tartar. But by several continental physicians the abstraction of blood is considered both unnecessary and hurtful. Thus Peschier advises on no account to draw blood; and Troussea observes, that bloodletting, far from aiding the action of emetic tartar, as Rasori, Laennec, and most practitioners, imagine, is, on the contrary, singularly injurious to the antiphlogistic influence of this medicine. Louis has published some numerical results of the treatment of inflammation of the lungs *by* bloodletting and by emetic tartar; from which it appears that this substance, given in large doses, where bloodletting appeared to.have no effect had a favourable action, and appeared to diminish the mortality. But he particularly states that bloodlctting must not be omitted.

Laennec's mode of using this salt, and which, with some slight modification, I believe to be the best, is the following:

Immediately after bleeding, give one grain of emetic tartar, dissolved in two ounces and a half of some mild fluid [cold weak infusion of orange flowers], sweetened with half an ounce of syrup of marshmallows: this is to be repeated every two hours for six times, and then suspended for seven or eight hours, if the symptoms are not urgent, or if there, be any inclination to sleep. Rut if the disease has already made progress, or if the oppression be great, or the head affected, continue the medicine until amendment takes place; and in severe cases increase the dose to two, or two and a half grains. The only modification in this plan, which I would venture to propose, is, to begin with a somewhat smaller dose (say one-third or one-half of a grain), and gradually increase it; for in consequence of the violent vomiting which one grain has sometimes produced, I have found patients positively refuse to continue the use of the medicine.

From *my* own experience, I should say that emetic tartar is nearly as serviceable when it causes moderate sickness and slight purging, as when it occasions no evacuation.

Laennec observes, that "in general the effect of emetic tartar is never more rapid, or more efficient, than when it gives rise to no evacuation; sometimes, however, its salutary operation is accompanied by a general perspiration. Although copious vomiting and purging are by no means desirable, on account of the debility and hurtful irritation of the intestinal canal which they may occasion, I have obtained remarkable cures in cases in which such evacuations have been very copious." A few drops of tincture of opium may be sometimes conjoined with the antimony, to check its action on the alimentary canal.

The attempts which have been made to explain the *modus medeni* of emetic tartar in pneumonia and other inflammatory diseases; are most unsatisfactory. Whilst almost every writer, even Broussais, admits its efficacy in inflammation, scarcely two agree in the view taken of the mode by which its good effects are produced, as the following statement proves: Rasori explains its operation according to the principles of the theory of contra-stimulus of which he may be regarded as the founder. He considers emetic tartar endowed with the power of directly diminishing the inflammatory stimulus, of destroying the diathesis, and of being, therefore, a real contra-stimulus. Broussais, Rouillaud, and Barbier ascribe its curative powers to its revulsive or derivative action on the gastro-intestinal membrane. Laennec thinks that it acts by increasing the activity of interstitial absorption. Fontaneilles supposes that the antiphlogistic effect depends on alterations in the composition of the blood. Eberle refers it to the sedative effects, first, on the nervous system, and consecutively on the heart and arteries. Teallier thinks that, like many other therapeutic agents, it influences the organism by concealed curative properties. Dr. Macartney regards it as a medicine diminishing the force of the circulation, by the nausea which it occasions. These examples are sufficient to show the unsatisfactory condition of our present knowledge as to the mode by which emetic tartar produces its curative effects. But this is no argument against the existence of remedial powers. Shall we deny the efficacy of bloodletting in inflammation, of mercury in syphilis, of cinchona in intermittents, of arsenic in lepra, of sulphur in scabies, of hydrocyanic acid in.gastrodynia, and of a host of other remedies, simply because we cannot account for their beneficial effects? The fact is, that in the present state of our knowledge we cannot explain the *modes medendi* of a large number of our best and most certain remedial means. (I have already offered some remarks on the modus medendi of liquefacients and resolvents at pp. 214 and 215.)

In *pleurisy* emetic tartar does not succeed so well as in inflammation of the substance of the lungs. "It, indeed, reduces speedily the inflammatory action," says Laennec, "but when the fever and. pain have ceased, the effusion does not always d.isappear more rapidly under the use of tartar emetic than without it." I have some,times conjoined. opium (always after copious bloodletting) with advantage. In *bronchitis* (both acute and chronic) it may be most usefully employed in conjunction with the usual antiphlogistic agents. In *rheumatism* (especially the kind called. *articular),* next to peripneumonia, emetic tartar has been found by some practitioners (especially by Laennec), more efficacious than in any other inflammatory affliction: the usual duration of the complaint, when treated by this remedy was found by Laennec to be seven or eight days. In muscular rheumatism it succeeds less perfectly. Synovial effusions (whether rheumatic or otherwise) have, in some cases given way rapidly to the use of emetic tartar. In *arachnitis,* Laennec has seen all the symptoms disappear, under the use of emetic tartar, in forty-eight hours. In three instances of acute hydrocephalus, all the symptoms disappeared in the same space of time. In *phlebitis,* in *inflammation of the mammae* occurring after delivery, in *ophthalmia,* and various other inflammatory affections, emetic tartar has been successfully employed as an antiphlogistic.

In continued fever, it is of considerable service. Mild cases are benefited by the use of small doses (as from one-sixteenth to one-fourth of a grain) as a diaphoretic. In the more severe form of this disease, accompanied with much vascular excitement, emetic tartar, in the dose of half a grain or a grain, may be usefully administered as an antiphlogistie; but its use should, in general, be preceded by bloodletting. In the advanced stages of typhus fever, accompanied with intense cerebral excitement, manifested by loss of sleep, delirium, &c., Dr. Graves has obtained most beneficial results from the use of emetic tartar and opium. The same combination has been employed with great success in delirium tremens, as well as in delirium of erysipelas, scarlatina, and measles, by Dr. Law.

Dr. Billing regards Asiatic cholera as being "like ague; not merely as regards its epidemic and miasmatic origin, but almost, if not altogether, an ague of a fresh type:" and. he depends much, in the treatment of it, on tartarized antimony with sulphate of magnesia. In a case of blue cholera he ordered two grains of emetic tartar and half an ounce of sulphate of magnesia in half a pint of water; a table-spoonful to be taken every half hour. The patient recovered.

Emetic tartar is one of our most valuable sudorifics, being oftentimes available when other agents of this class are inadmissible: for example, when we are desirous of producing diaphoresis, in fevers and other diseases which are accompanied with preternatural vascular action about the head, the use of opiate sudorifics (as the compound ipecacunnha powder) is objectionable; whereas emetic tartar may be employed with safety, since it has no tendency to increase disorder of the nervous system, but to reduce cerebral excitement. On the other hand, when much gastric or intestinal irritation is present, the narcotic sudorifics are generally to be preferred to antimony.

As an expectorant, in various pulmonary affections, small doses of this salt are frequently employed with advantage.

In some spasmodic complaints, the use of it has been followed, in the few instances in which it has been tried, with good effects. In *apoplexy, it* has been employed to depress cerebral vascular action, but its tendency to occasion vomiting renders it objectionable.

The internal employment of emetic tartar in syphilis has been recently advocated by Mr. Smee.

As a local irritant, applied to the skin, it may be employed in the form of aqueous solution, ointment, or plaster. It is used in the same case as vesicatories, over which it has the advantage of not affecting the urino-genital organs. When it is desirable to keep up long-continued irritatiou, blisters are in some cases preferable.

In *chronic diseases of the chest* it is used with the greatest advantage. I have found it much more serviceable than blisters. I frequently direct one part of the chest to be rubbed until the eruption is produced; and then, after the interval of a day or two, another part; thus keeping up irritation by a succession of applications to different parts of the chest for several months. In this way it is most serviceable in chronic catarrhs, peripneumonies, aud pleurisies. Even in lingering phthisis I have seen the cough and pain alleviated by the occasional use of antimonial frictions. The objections to its use is the painful character of the eruptions.

In w*hooping-cough* it is also serviceable. Autenrieth recommended it as a means of diminishing the frequency of the paroxysms and the violence of the cough. In *laryngitis* it is occasionally of great service; as also in various *operations of the joints,* especially chronic inflammation of the capsular ligament, or of the synovial membrane, hydrops articuli, particularly when connected with inflammation, and tumours of various kinds about the joints. In *tic douloireux'* it has also been employed with benefit. In the *paralysis* of children, the region of the spine should be rubbed with the ointment. Its effects are most beneficial, especially when one leg only is affected. It is sometimes necessary to keep an eruption out for many weeks. In *hysteria,* the same application to the spine has been found serviceable.

A *stimulating* wash, composed of one scruple of tartar emetic to an ounce of water, was proposed by the late Sir William Blizard, in the year 1787, to cleanse foul ulcers, repress fungous growths and venereal warts, and as an application to tinea capitis. A weak solution (as half a grain to the ounce of water) has been employed as a stimulant in chronic ophthalmia, and in spots on the cornea.

Administration.– The-dose of emetic tartar, *in substance,* is, as a diaphoretic and expectorant, one-twelfth to one-sixth of a grain: as a nauseant, from one-fourth to one-half a grain; as an emetic, from 1 to 2 grains; as an antiphlogistic, from one-half a grain to 3 or 4 grains. This salt is, however, rarely employed in substance. Sometimes a grain of it, mixed with ten or fifteen grains of powdered ipecacuanha, is employed as an emetic. A mixture of one grain with sixteen grains of sulphate of potash may be employed, in doses of from two to four grains, as a substitute for antimonial powder, to promote diaphoresis.

In *solution,* it is commonly employed as an expectorant, diaphoretic, nauseant, or emetic in the form of antimonial wine. When used as an antiphlogistic, an aqueous solution of greater strength may be administered: it should be made with boiling distilled water in a glass vessel (as a Florence flask).

For external use, emetic tartar is employed in the form of *liniment, ointment,* or *plaster.* A saturated solution is a very useful liniment: it is prepared by pouring an ounce and a half of boiling water over a drachm of emetic tartar, and allowing the solution to stand till cold. In many cases it will be found preferable to the ointment; being the mildest, least painful, and cleanest. Another mode of employing emetic tartar externally is by sprinkling from ten grains to a drachm of the salt in fine powder over a Burgundy pitch plaster.

Bruce A. Evans, M.D.

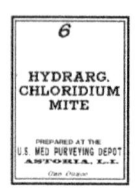

```
    6
HYDRARG.
CHLORIDIUM
   MITE
PREPARED AT THE
U.S. MED PURVEYING DEPOT
  ASTORIA, L.I.
```

Hydrargyri Chloridium Mite (Calomel
Heavy, light buff or ivory color powder

(Use has been documented since 1497)

   This is formulated as a mild form of mercury ("mite"). It is insoluble, and is administered in syrup or molasses or as a pill combined with gum arabic and sugar. It produces all of the effects of mercury on the system, and is usually the best form for internal use, being mild yet certain in its action. In small doses (up to ¼ grain) it has a peculiarly specific effect on inflammatory disease of unknown mechanism (alterative) without other effects. In larger doses it is mildly cathartic, and it also increases secretions — especially salivation, which may benefit the condition of the tongue, although prolonged use causes ulcers and eventually tissue destruction in the mouth. To prevent this, the medication should not be used after increased salivation and the usually accompanying fetid breath appear. This medication is most useful for treating inflammation after the first few days of acute inflammation have been treated by other means (purging, use of **tarter emetic**, or, less commonly now, bleeding), or when inflammation is present in a low disease (such as typhoid) in which the usual depleting methods would be dangerous and inappropriate. Larger doses cause purging. Some feel it increases bile secretion — this has been disproved in experiments using dogs. The dose is ½ grain to two grains, every evening or every other evening. A laxative should be given on the second day if the bowels have not moved. The dose may be divided and given every few hours if the stomach or bowels are irritable.

Modern Perspective:

Mercury Chloride was felt to be a "milder" form of mercury; however, we know now that such mercury salts, unlike elemental mercury, are readily absorbed from the gut into the body, and hence are even more toxic.

Toxicity information: A highly toxic compound. 30 to 40 mg. per kg. of body weight may well be fatal if not vomited. Three days after ingestion, inflammation of the mouth, severe diarrhea, and kidney dysfunction appear. Salivation is stimulated, and is in fact one of the routes of excretion. Complete kidney failure may occur.

The reasons for the faith in the healing powers of mercury, in its various forms, is unclear. Its effect of stimulation of salivation may have been seen to "benefit" the appearance of a tongue taking on a foul aspect secondary to fever, dehydration, and mouth breathing. 19th century (and earlier) doctors gave great weight to the diagnostic value of the appearance of the tongue, and lacking knowledge of almost any disease cause, concentrated on medications which returned some or one of the patient's observed abnormalities towards the "natural state". At one point it was felt to increase the bile flow, but this had been disproven by animal experiments by the 1850s. It also was, at best, an uncertain and unreliable laxative. There was a centuries-long tradition of treating venereal disease with mercury: it may have had some beneficial effect but clearly also had long-term toxicity.

In the end, the medication's largely imagined beneficial effect on inflammatory disease was classified as an "alterative" effect - "we think it helps but we don't know how or why".

By the 1860s some physicians recognized the harm done to patients by (over)use of mercurial medications, including gangrene (essentially rotting) of the tissues of the gums and mouth with chronic use. William Hammond, the controversial Federal Surgeon General, tried to ban calomel from government surgeon's use and was literally run off the job following the outrage of more traditional practitioners (although the excuse on which he was dismissed was formally unrelated to that action).

From a modern perspective, this drug was not accomplishing any good for the patients.

Period Reference:

The Elements of Materia Medica and Therapeutics – Jonathan Pereira, M.D. (Blanchard and Lee, Philadelphia, 1852) on the uses and administration of:

Uses – Calomel is very frequently used as an *alterative,* in glandular affections, chronic skin diseases, and disordered conditions of the digestive organs, more particularly in those cases connected with hepatic derangement. For this purpose it is usually taken in. combination with other alteratives, as in the well-known Plummer's pill, which I shall presently notice.

It is very frequently employed as a *purgative,* though on account of the uncertainty of its cathartic effects, it is seldom given alone; generally in combination with other drastic purgatives – such as jalap, scammony, compound extract of colocynth, &c., whose activity it very much promotes. We employ it for this purpose when we are desirous of relieving affections of other organs, on the principle of counter-irritation. Thus in threatened apoplexy, in mental disorders, in dropsical affections, and in chronic diseases of the akin. In torpid conditions of the bowels, where it is necessary to use powerful cathartics to produce alvine evacuations, as in paralytic affections, it is advantageously combined with other purgatives. Sometimes we use it to promote the biliary secretion – as in jaundice and other affections of the liver, in chronic skin diseases, and. in various disordered conditions of the alimentary canal not accompanied by inflammation. Moreover, in the various diseases of children requiring the use of purgatives, it is generally considered to be very useful; and its being devoid of taste is of course an advantage.

As a *sedative* it has been administered in yellow fever, spasmodic or malignant cholera, dysentery, and liver affections. Dr. Griflin asserts that calomel proved a most successful medicine in cholera, controlling or arresting its progress in 84 cases out of 100, when administered while the pulse was perceptible at the wrist; but that, on the contrary, it proved detrimental when given in collapse. The practice was tested in 1,448 eases. The dose was from one to two scruples every hour or half-hour.

As a *sialagogue,* it may be used in the cases in which I have already stated that mercurials generally are employed: with the view of preventing irritation of the alimentary canal, it is usually given in combination with opium, unless the existence of some affection of the nervous system contra,indicates the use of narcotics. This combination is employed in peripneumonia, pleuritis, croup, laryngitis, hepa.titis, enteritis, and. other inflammatory diseases: in fever, syphilis, chronic visceral diseases, &c.

Calomel is frequently combined with other medicines, to increase their effects; as with squills) to produce *diuresis* in dropsy; or, with antimonials to promote *diaphoresis.*

As an *anthelmintic,* it is in frequent use, and forms one of the active ingredients of many of the nostrums sold for worms; though it does not appear to have any specific iufluence over parasitic animals.

The *local uses* of calomel are numerous. In diseases of the Schneiderian membrane, it is applied as a snuff. It is sometimes blown into the eye to remove spots on the cornea. Dr. Pricke has used it with great success in chronic cases of rheumatic, catarrhal, and scrofulous ophthalmia; but in two instances bad consequences resulted from its use. It is sometimes suspended in thick mucilage, and. used as a gargle in venereal sore-throat, or injected into the urethra in blennorrhea. Now and then it is used as a substitute for cinnabar in fumigation. As a local application, in the form of ointment, calomel is one of the most useful remedies we possess for the cure of several forms of chronic skin diseases.

Administration– When used as an *alterative, it* is given in doses of from half a grain to a grain, frequently combined with oxysulphuret of antimony (as in *Plummer's pill)* or antimonial powder, and repeated every, or every other night; a mild saline laxative being given the following morning. As a *purgative,* from two to five grains are given usually in combination with, or followed by, the use of other purgatives, especially jalap, senna, scammony, or colocynth. As a *sialagogue,* it is exhibited in doses of one to three or four grains, generally combined with opium or Rover's powder, twice or thrice a day. As a *sedative,* the dose is from 'a scruple to half a drachm or more. Biett has sometimes employed it as an *errhine,* in syphilitic eruptions. It is mixed with some inert powder, and given to the extent of from 8 to 20 grains daily. The use of acids with calomel frequently occasions griping. Calomel is most extensively employed in the diseases of children, and may be given to them in as large or proportionally larger doses than to adults. Salivation is a rare occurrence in them: indeed, Mr. Colles asserts that mercury *never* produces ptyalism, or swelling or ulceration of the gums, in infants; but this is an error (see *ante*, p. 7.99).

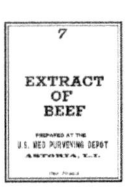

Extract of Beef
Brownish powder

Diet is an important treatment in various disease states. In general, foods of high nutritive value are used to build up a debilitated patient as components of a high - restorative or strengthening - diet. They should not be used, however, in patients with diseases characterized by overexcitement of the system - the sthenic or inflammatory diseases accompanied by rapid and forceful pulse, high fever, and so on - since this would essentially add fuel to the fire. These latter would be treated with a low diet made up of small amounts of food mainly of vegetable origin.

Beef tea made of beef extract heated in water is used to fortify and strengthen in chronic diarrhea or dysentery, or in other low or aesthenic diseases or debilitated state after trauma or wounds, as part of a restorative diet. It should be used with caution in chronic diarrhea or dysentery, as a feeble digestive system may not tolerate it. In such cases, diets rich in milk (**Milk, Condensed**) or eggs, which are easier on the digestion, are preferred.

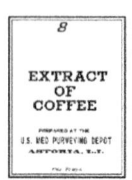

Extract of Coffee
Brownish powder

Coffee owes its stimulant properties to caffeine, and perhaps to a tannin component. Its effect differs from **Tea, Black** mainly in degree, being richer in caffeine than that substance. It is prepared by adding the powder to warm water. It is used as a mild to moderate stimulant in low or aesthenic diseases such as typhoid fever, especially when the patient is overly sleepy. It acts as a stimulant to the brain without a marked effect on the frequency or force of the pulse. Interestingly, it is also often useful, in those not inured to its effects through frequent use, in treating a sick headache.

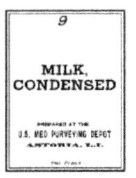

Milk, Condensed

A nutrient especially useful in bowel disorders, when a nutritive diet is demanded but meat products are poorly tolerated.

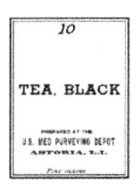

Tea, Black —
dark brown leaves

This is used as stimulant in low or asthenic diseases, similarly to **Extract of Coffee**. It is often more palatable and easier on the stomach than coffee, with similar but often milder effects. It is prepared as an infusion with hot water.

Bruce A. Evans, M.D.

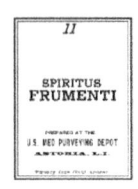

Spiritus Frumenti (whiskey)

Alcohol in any form is a strong stimulant of the brain as well as the circulation, causing exhilaration and a stronger, more forceful pulse. It is therefore used as a as stimulant in low or aesthenic diseases, and especially as stimulant to treat collapse after severe trauma or wounds. It is useful in the low or asthenic febrile diseases such as typhoid. However, it is also used in the late stages of initially sthenic inflammatory disease when debilitation and collapse occur, especially when abscess formation or suppuration drains the stength of the patient. Examples of this latter use include the late stage of pneumonia, erysipelas, suppuration in the joints, and gangrene. This product is derived from the distillation of grain (usually rye) fermentation, and is used to deliver a substantial dose of alcohol in a small amount of liquid.

Modern Perspective:

It is interesting, but not surprising, that this bottle is the largest in the set. The main use of whiskey, as a stimulant, for the civil war surgeon was to treat the collapse involved with severe trauma, such as a significant wound.

The concept of shock, representing a circulatory impairment progressing to collapse caused by blood loss was not recognized. Currently such trauma is treated immediately, even on the battlefield, by the infusion of fluids directly into the veins to

The Practice of Civil War Medicine and Surgery

support the circulation. Lacking both the physiologic knowledge and the availability of sterile fluids and a means of introducing them, the civil war surgeon used such "stimulants".

It is of interest that the medical reports of the time did include a report from India in which a person in the last stages of collapse from cholera - which kills due to profuse diarrhea leading to dehydration and shock - was marvelously revived by the infusion into the vein of a water and salt solution. Unfortunately, the patient died 24 hours later from what was undoubtably an overwhelming blood infection brought on by the non-sterile infusion.

The "stimulant" role of alcoholic products had, of course, a long tradition behind it. Unfortunately, the actual effects - other than whatever benefit to the feeling of well-being and mild pain relief intoxication may have provided - are more depressant in nature and had no beneficial, and more probably a detrimental, physiologic effect on the wounded soldier.

The presence of this bottle in the supply sets did certainly have the effect of making medical supplies a point of attention for looting troops of either side. The Latin name on the bottle would have been of little protection.

One and a half to two pints taken quickly are a potentially fatal dose - this dose was not approached in normal battlefield use.

Period Reference:

The Elements of Materia Medica and Therapeutics – Jonathan Pereira, M.D. (Blanchard and Lee, Philadelphia, 1852) on the uses and administration of:
Ardent Spirits (Whiskey)

Uses.– Ardent Spirits are employed both for medicinal and pharmaceutical purposes.

1. Medicinal Uses.– Spirit is used both internally and externally: –

a. **Internally**.– Spirit of wine is rarely administered internally; for when ardent spirit is indicated, Brandy, Gin, or Whiskey, is generally employed. The separate uses of each of these will be noticed presently; at present, therefore, I shall confine myself to some general remarks on the internal employment of spirit. I may observe, however, that Brandy is the ardent spirit usually administered for medicinal purposes; and, unless otherwise stated, is the spirit referred to in the following observations. As a *stomachic stimulant,:* spirit is employed to relieve spasmodic pains and flatulency, to check vomiting (especially sea-sickness), and to give temporary relief in some cases of indigestion, attended with pain after taking food. As a *stimulant and restorative,* it is given with considerable advantage in the latter stages of fever. As a *powerful excitant,* it is used to support the vital powers, to prevent fainting during a tedious operation, to relieve syncope and languor, and to assist the restoration of patients from a state of suspended animation. In *delirium tremens,* it is not always advisable to leave off the employment of spirituous liquors at once, since the sudden withdrawal of .the long accustomed stimulus may be attended with fatal consequences. In such cases, it is advisable to allow, temporarily, to the patient the moderate use of the particular kind of spirit which he has been in the habit of employing. In p*oisoninp by foxglove and tobacco,* spirit and ammonia are used to rouse the action of the heart. In *mild cases of diarrhea,,* attended with griping pain, but unaccompanied by any inflammatory symptoms, a small quantity of spirit and water, taken warm, with nutmeg, is often a mpst efficacious remedy.

b. **Externally**.– Ardent spirits are used externally for several purposes, of which the following are the principal: As a *styptic,* to restrain hemorrhage from weak and relaxed parts. It proves efficacious in two ways; it coagulates the blood by its chemical influence on the liquid, albumen, and fibrin, and it causes the contraction of the mouths of the bleeding vessels by its stimulant and astringent qualities.

Sponge or soft linen, soaked in spirit and water, has been applied to the mouth of the uterus in uterine hemorrhage. *Spirit is employed to harden the cuticle over tender and delicate parts.* Thus, brandy is sometimes applied to the nipples, several weeks before delivery, in order to prevent the production of sore nipples from suckling in individuals predisposed to it. Spirit is also applied to the feet, when the skin is readily blistered by walking. The efficacy of spirit, in hardening the cuticle, depends, in part, on its chemical influence. Spirit gargles have been found. serviceable in checking the tendency to inflammation and swelling of the tonsils. As *a stimulant application,* warm rectified spirit has been applied to burned or scalded parts, on the principles laid down for the treatment of these cases by Dr. Kentish. Properly diluted, spirit has been employed as a wash in *various skin diseases,* and *in ulcers of bed-ridden persons,* and as a *collyrium in* chronic ophthalmia. *Frictions with rectified spirits* have been used in the abdominal region, to promote labour pains; on the chest, to excite the action of the heart, in fainting or suspended animation; on the hypogastric region, to stimulate the bladder, when retention of urine depends on inertia, or a paralytic condition of this viscus; on various parts of the body, to relieve the pain arising from bruises, or to stimulate paralyzed. parts. *The inhalation of the vapour of rectified spirit* has been recommended to relieve the irritation produced by the inspiration of chlorine; but I have tried the practice on myself without benefit.The readiest mode of effecting it is to drop some spirit on a lump of sugar, and hold this in the mouth during inspiration.

Diluted spirit has been used as *an injection for the radical cure of hydrocele.* A mixture of wine and water, however, is commonly employed in this country.

S*pirit has been used to form cold lotions. As* the efficacy of it depends on its evaporation, it should be applied by means of a single layer of linen, and not by a compress. Evaporating lotions are applied to the head in cephalalgia, in phrenitis, in fever, in poisoning by opium, Re.; to fractures of the extremities; to parts affected with erysipelatous inflammations, &c.

Antidotes.– The first object in the treatment of poisoning by spirituous liquors is to evacuate the contents of the stomach. This is best effected by the stomach- pump; emetics being frequently unsuccessful. Stimulants are then to be employed: the most effectual are the injection of cold water into the ears, cold affusion to the head and neck, warmth to the extremities, when these are cold, and the internal use either of ammonia or of the solution of the acetate of ammonia, both of which agents have been found useful in relieving stupor. The cerebral congestion often requires the cautious employment of local bloodletting and the application of cold to the head. If the patient appear to be dying from paralysis of the respiratory muscles, artificial respiration should be effected; if from closure of the larynx, tracheotomy may be performed.

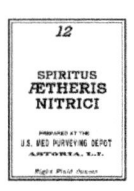

Spiritus Ætheris Nitrici (sweet spirit of nitre) -
Colorless or yellowish liquid; peculiar odor like ripe apples
(Use documented since the 15th century or earlier)

This medication is often used together with **Antimonii et Potassæ Tartras** for fever, increasing the perspiration produced (diaphoretic effect) and also causing increased urine (diuretic effect) in larger doses up to 2 teaspoons. This relieves the hot dry skin and scanty urine often accompanying febrile disease. In addition, it benefits the underlying inflammation by depleting the blood of watery fluid and causing action at the skin, withdrawing system energy from the inflammation (revulsive action). It is also useful for nausea. Used alone, it is not a particularly powerful diuretic or diaphoretic, but because it is a nervous stimulant without sedative effect on the circulation, it is particularly useful when such effect on the circulation must be avoided but nervous stimulation is warranted, as in typhoid disease. 30 minims in a full glass of cold water every two to four hours is the dose for increasing sweating; 1 fluidrachm should be used to increase urination.

Modern Perspective:

Nitrates such as this cause flushing, headache, perspiration, and the (irreversible) formation of a form of hemoglobin which is an ineffective oxygen carrier (methemaglobin). Therefore, cyanosis (blue tinge to lips, other mucous membranes, nailbeds, etc.) may result.

The perspiration induced was felt to benefit a feverish, dehydrated, and therefore dry-skinned sick patient by returning the skin towards the "natural state". This was a result of being in a position of treating symptoms only, given the lack of knowledge of the underlying cause of the disease being treated, most of which were due to as yet unidentified micro-organisms.

From a modern point of view, this treatment accomplishes little and may increase the patient's dehydration.

Period Reference:

The Elements of Materia Medica and Therapeutics – Jonathan Pereira, M.D. (Blanchard and Lee, Philadelphia, 1852) on the uses and administration of:
Sweet Spirit of Nitre

Uses.– It is employed as a diuretic in some disorders of children, and in mild dropsical complaints, as in the anasarca which follows scarlatina. It is given in conjunction with squills, acetate or nitrate of potash, or foxglove. As a refrigrant and diaphoretic, it is used in febrile complaints in combination with the acetate of ammonia and emetic tartar. As a carminative, it is frequently useful in relieving flatulence and allaying nausea. On account of its volatility, it may be applied to produce cold by its evaporation. Spirit dealers employ it as a flavouring ingredient.

Administration.– The usual dose of this liquid, in febrile cases, is one-half to two fluiddrachm or three fluiddrachm. When we wish it to act as a diuretic, it should be given in large doses, as two or three teaspoonfuls.

Antidotes.– In poisoning by the inhalation of the vapour of this compound, the treatment will be the same as that described for poisoning by carbonic acid gas.

Bruce A. Evans, M.D.

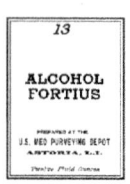

```
13
ALCOHOL
FORTIUS

PREPARED AT THE
U.S. MED PURVEYING DEPOT
ASTORIA, N.Y.
```

Alcohol, Fortius (strong alcohol)

This form of alcohol, considerably purer than the distilled ardent spirits such as **Spiritus Frumenti**, is not meant for internal use. It is the strongest form of alcohol that can be produced by simple distillation. It is used mainly to prepare tinctures of substances not soluble in water. It is also used on the skin, wet upon a single layer of linen, to provide local cooling and blood vessel constriction through the evaporative effect to treat local inflammation. Diluted, it can be used internally for stimulation if no alternative is available. Thus depending on the approach, it may be used for systemic stimulation, local sedation, or in the preparation of liquid forms of other medications for systemic use.

Modern Perspective:

*This form of alcohol, considerably purer than the distilled ardent spirits usch as **Spiritus Frumenti**, is not meant for internal use. It is the strongest form of alcohol that can be produced by simple distillation. It is used mainly to prepare tinctures of substances not soluble in water. It is also used on the skin, wet upon a single layer of linen, to provide local cooling and blood vessel constriction through the evaporative effect to treat local inflammation. Diluted, it can be used internally for stimulation if no alternative is available. Thus depending on the approach, it may be used for systemic stimulation, local* *sedation, or in the preparation of liquid forms of other medications for systemic use.*

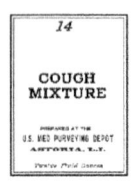

Cough Mixture

This is a compounded mixture consisting of Syrup of Squills (for expectorant effect) and Camphorated Tincture of Opium (for cough suppression), four fluid ounces each, and two fluid drachms of Fluid Extract of Ipecacuanha (for expectorant and anti-inflammatory effect). It is used for acute or chronic cough.

Modern Perspective:

The addition of the syrup of squills and the non-emetic dose of ipecac to this mixture, dictated by anti-inflammatory theory, add nothing to its effect. The cough suppressant effect is due entirely to the opium.

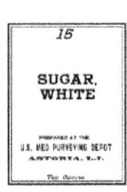

Sugar, White -
White crystalline grains

Sugar may be used as strengthening nutrient in low or aesthenic diseases. It may also be used as antiseptic to treat mortification of wounds. However, it is mainly used to combine with water to produce syrups as a vehicle for other medications, to improve the cohesiveness of pills, or to flavor bitter or unpleasant tasting medication to secure improved compliance from the patient for a necessary course of treatment.

Bruce A. Evans, M.D.

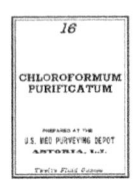

Chloroformum Purificatum (Pure Chloroform) -
Colorless liquid

This is used as an anesthetic, with 2 fluidrachms soaked into a towel arranged into a cone and the base then held over the nose and mouth, or a lesser amount dripped slowly onto a linen rag lying over the mouth and nose. It does not seem to have the extent of unfortunate initial stimulation of ether used for an anesthetic, and its vapors are less flammable, allowing surgery to proceed by lantern light.

Modern Perspective:

Chloroform is an effective operative anesthetic, and probably safer in the war era than ether due to a lesser flammability than ether which is very explosive, a definite weakness in an era of open flames for illumination. Chloroform is also more potent than either, and subjects therefore move more quickly through the initial excitement phase present during induction than with ether anesthesia. The main toxicity preventing modern use is cardiac irritability; the relative safety during the civil war era likely resulted from the light levels of anesthesia and the relatively brief duration of the procedures.

Period Reference:

The Practice of Civil War Medicine and Surgery
The Elements of Materia Medica and Therapeutics – Jonathan Pereira, M.D. (Blanchard and Lee, Philadelphia, 1852) on the uses and administration of:

Physiological Effects.– In medicinal doses, chloroform is a stimulant, sedative, antispasmodic, and anesthetic. In large doses, it causes profound coma and death. In man, it has been observed to cause excessive depression of the heart's action, and in persons affected with disease of this organ, ordinary doses have on several occasions proved fatal.

Administration.– Chloroform is seldom taken as a liquid; the dose is from five to ten minima, mixed with water and a little mucilage. The dose for inhalation of the vapour is from one to three drachms. Dr. Simpson, however, has used as much as eight fluidounces in thirteen hours, in a case of labour. Its administration requires great care, and some experience on the part of the practitioner.

Uses.– Chloroform is now chiefly used as an agent for obtaining insensibility to pain during operations, and is therefore to be regarded more especially as an adjuvant to surgery. Before noticing the general history of its application in the above-mentioned manner, it may be well to state that it has also been used with advantage as a substitute for the ethers, and found to possess equal efficacy as a stimulant and antispasmodic. The form in which it has been ordinarily exhibited, is in admixture with rectified spirit; and it is sold in the shops in this diluted condition under the name of chloric ether. This is a most improper appellation, inasmuch as the term chloric ether is understood by chemists to refer to an oil-like fluid, formed by the reaction of chlorine upon olefiant gas (see page 980). This solution of chloroform is, for the most part, made by adding one part of that fluid to nine parts of rectfied spirit; the dose for an adult being from twenty minima to forty two or three times a day. It may be used as a substitute for the sulphuric ether in all cases requiring an anti-spasmodic and stimulant remedy; and as its flavour is preferred by most persons to that of the ethereal preparations, it may be advantageously prescribed where abjuration is made to the latter form of stimulant.

Bruce A. Evans, M.D.

With respect to the mode of using chloroform as an anesthetic agent, by introducing it into the circulation during the respiratory process, experience has shown that this can only be done with any degree of safety by allowing the vapour to be admixed with atmospheric air in considerable proportion before it is taken into the lungs. This is effected. by a variety of contrivances. The principle on which the earlier instruments for inhaling were constructed, was to close the nasal aperture by a spring clasp, and so to insure the admission of the atmospheric air merely to the extent it might please the operator to permit by the mouth. The best instruments now in use are, however, constructed so as to allow the vapour to pass both by the nose and the mouth into the lungs, the patient being made to breathe through a mask. The form recommended by Dr. Snow, who has paid great attention to this subject, is figured in the accompanying woodcut, for which we are indebted to Dr. Snow. The mask is of simple construction, and is fixed to an inhaler of Dr. Snow's invention, which enables the operator to adjust the proportion of chloroform vapour to atmospheric air. The directions for use, which are appended to the description of the inhaler, will enable the reader at once to understand the principle of its action. If from two to three drachms of chloroform be used, the air respired will contain from five to six per cent. of vapour of chloroform; and this is cnnsidered by Dr. Snow to be a safe proportion.

The important observations made by Dr. Snow, with respect to the action of chloroform on the lower animals, as well as the facts he has collectecl with regard to the deaths which have taken place in the human subject while chloroform was being inhaled, seem to have determined the following points very satisfactorily: –

1stly. Chloroform vapour, if it be inhaled in large proportion with atmospheric air, destroys life by paralyzing the heart.

2dly. In smaller proportions, but long continued, it produces death apparently by the brain, and by interfering with the respiratory function. In such cases the heart is found to beat after respiration has ceased.

3dly. Chloroform vapour, if it be blown upon the heart, paralyzes it immediately.

4thly. Atmospheric air; loaded with from 4 to 5, or even 6 per cent. of chloroform vapour, may be safely administered, inasmuch as that mixture will not act directly upon the heart, but will give timely notice of its increasing effects in modifying the normal discharge of the functions of life. The average time occupied in producing insensibility is from three to four minutes.

5thly. The proportion of as much as from 8 to 10 per cent. of vapour of chloroform to atmospheric air is a dangerous mixture, as it suddenly charges the blood going into the heart with a poison capable of acting directly on that organ.

From the above statement it would appear probable that many, if not all; the deaths which have so unfortunately occurred from the use of chloroform, have been the result of the too sudden administration of the vapour, and that in many cases much more than that quantity which caused dissolution might have been safely taken, had it been administered in a more diluted form.

To the experience of Dr. Snow, and the solid nature of his reasoning on this subject, we find opposed many very bold statements. Thus it has been recommended as the safest plan, to give the chloroform in large doses at once, and bring about anesthesia as rapidly as can be effected. It is scarcely possible, however, after due consideration, to come to any other conclusion than that there has been more good luck than good management attending the practice of those gentlemen who act in direct opposition to rules laid down in accordance with the best results of careful experiment and accurate reasoning. Notwithstanding, however, that the knowledge we now possess may enable us, with due care, to protect from death healthy persons who inhale chloroform, it must be remembered that fatal cases must be expected in certain diseased conditions, even when every precaution has been taken. Thus it cannot be doubted, that where the heart is affected either with extensive disease of its component structures or of its valvular appliances, the dose of chloroform which might be perfectly safe in health may in such cases produce a fatal result. This remark especially applies where the heart is weakened either by fatty degeneration or fatty deposit, or where atrophy of its tissue and thinning of the walls of the organ have, to any considerable extent, lessened its muscular power. It unfortunately happens, too, that these conditions, and especially the former, are not always easily ascertainable during life. Again, we may expect that lesion of the brain, of an obscure character, may sometimes render the inhalation hazardous.

On the whole, then, even with every precaution, it would seem that to give chloroform to induce anesthesia, is to introduce an additional element of danger during an operation. Experience has shown that this amount of danger is but very small; and therefore, when every care is taken, and no obvious disease can be detected in the internal organs of the patient, it may sometimes be justifiable to *re*commend. the inhalation of chloroform, in order to secure the patient from suffering.

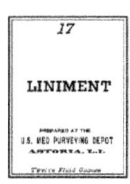

Liniment —
white syrupy liquid

This substance is used as emollient application and to provide a mild counter-stimulation when applied externally to sooth irritated areas: It is compounded of equal parts Water of Ammonia, Oil of Turpentine, and Olive Oil.

Modern Perspective:

This is an essentially non-toxic substance without significant medical activity.

Bruce A. Evans, M.D.

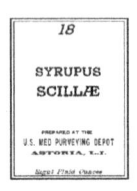

```
18
SYRUPUS
SCILLÆ
PREPARED AT THE
U.S. MED PURVEYING DEPOT
ASTORIA, L.I.
```

Syrupus Scillæ (syrup of squill) -
White or yellowish-white syrup

In doses greater than 1 fluidrachm, this is a harsh emetic and purgative. Due to this harshness, it is little used. It has some expectorant activity to help clear chronic cough.

Modern Perspective:

It is well that this substance causes explosive vomiting and diarrhea, since if retained it has significant heart and central nervous system toxicity.

The magnitude of the purgative effect can be judged from the contemporary view that this drug was probably too harsh to use, when the use of other extremely energetic emetics and purgatives was routine.

Period Reference:

The Elements of Materia Medica and Therapeutics – Jonathan Pereira, M.D. (Blanchard and Lee, Philadelphia, 1852) on the uses and administration of:
Squill

Uses.– The principal uses of squill are those of an emetic, diuretic, and expectorant.

1. *As a diuretic in dropsies.–* It is applicable to those cases of dropsy requiring the use of stimulating or acrid diuretics, and, is improper in inflammatory cases. It is an unfit remedy for dropsy complicated with

granular kidney or vesical irritation; but when these conditions are not present, it is adapted. for torpid. leucophlegmatic subjects. Hence, it is more serviceable in anasarca than in either ascites or hydrothorax. It should be given so as to excite a slight degree of nausea (not vomiting), as recommended by Van Swieten. By this means its absorption is promoted. The acetate or bitartrate of potash may be conjoined. Calomel is usually regarded as a good adjunct for promoting the diuretic influence of squill. When it does not purge it is beneficial, but its tendency to affect the bowels is an objection to its use.

2. As an expectorant in chronic pulmonary affections admitting of the use of a substance stimulating the capillary vessels of the bronchial membrane. Thus, in chronic catarrh, humid asthma, and winter cough, it is often employed with considerable benefit. It is of course improper in all acute cases accompanied with inflammation or febrile disorder. In old persons it is often combined with the *tincfura camphor' combosita,* and with good effect. The oxymel or syrup of squill may be given to relieve troublesome chronic coughs in children.

3. As *an emetic,* it is occasionally used in affections of the organs of respiration requiring or admitting of the use of vomits. Thus, the oxymel is given, with the view of creating sickness and promoting expectoration, to children affected. with hooping-cough; and sometimes, though with less propriety, in mild cases of croup. The great objection to its use is the uncertainty of its operation: in one case it will hardly excite nausea, in another it causes violent vomiting. Furthermore, it is of course highly objectionable as an emetic for delicate children with irritable stomachs, on account of its acrid properties, and the irritation it is capable, in these cases, of setting up.

Administration.– The following are the preparations of squills usually employed: –

SYRUPUS SCILLAE COMPOSITUS , *U.S.; Compound Syrup of Squill; Hive Syrup* –

Take of Squill bruised, Senega bruised, each four ounces; Tartrate of Antimony and Potassa forty-eight grains; Water four pints; Sugar three pounds and a half. Pour the water upon the squill and senega, and having boiled to one-half, strain, and add the sugar; then evaporate to three pints, and, while the syrup is still hot, dissolve in it the tartrate of antimony and potassa. Another mode of preparation is, take of Squill in coarse powder, Senega in coarse powder, each four ounces; Tartrate of Antimony and Potassa forty-eight grains; Alcohol half a pint; Water a sufficient quantity; Sugar three pounds and a half. Mix the alcohol with two pints and a half of water, and macerate the squill and senega in the mixture for twenty-four hours. Put the whole in an apparatus for displacement, aud' add. as nuch water as may be necessary to make the altered liquor amount to three pints. Boil the liquor for a few minutes, evaporate to one-half, and strain; then add the sugar and evaporate until the resulting syrup measures three pints. Lastly, dissolve the tartrate of antimony and potassa in the syrup, while it is still hot.

This preparation is a modification of that made according to the formula given

by Dr. J. R. Coxe, and which goes by the name of *Coxe's Hive Syrup.* In the former editions of the Pharmacopoeia, the formula of Dr. Coxe was adopted; and as honey was substituted for sugar, it had the officinal name of *Mel Scillae compositum.* The formula above cited authorizes the substitution of sugar for honey, as it is less liable, when prepared as directed, to undergo fermentation – a great desideratum in hot weather. There is no difference between the proportions of the ingredients, so that an equal strength of the two preparations is obtained by both. The latter was introduced in accordance with the recommendation of the Committee of Revision of the Philadelphia College of Pharmacy.

This preparation combines the advantages of squill, senega, and tartarized antimony, and is an exceedingly active preparation. In sufficient doses, it operates upon the stomach, producing free vomiting and expectoration. It is used at the commencement of croup, hooping-cough, and catarrhal affections in children, with the view to its evacuant impression. In the inflammatory stages, as an expectorant and nauseant, it may also be employed with advantage, in reduced doses. The dose is from 10 drops to a fluiddrachm, according to the age of the child, repeated every ten or fifteen minutes until it pukes. As an expectorant for adults, the dose is 20 to 30 drops.

Antidote.– No antidote is known. The first object, therefore, in a case of poisoning, is to evacuate the stomach; the second, to allay the inflammatory symptoms which may supervene.

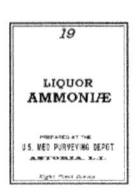

Liquor Ammoniæ (ammonia water) —
colorless liquid

Sufficiently diluted this is a prompt and powerful agent for reddening, blistering, or scarring the skin in inflammatory affections (depending on the degree of dilution and the contact time) in which a strong and prompt counter-irritation is required, including various neuralgic, gouty, rheumatic, or spasmodic disorders. It is applied with stupes, created by soaking linen strips and laying them over a suitable skin area.

Modern Perspective:

This irritative substance was used to provoke an inflammatory reaction on the skin when applied in various ways and mixed with various adherent substance. The degree of irritation and inflammation induced could be varied based on the amount of dilution of the substance. It produces a more energetic response than capsicum.

The presumed benefits of that reaction, in reducing pathologic inflammation in a contiguous area ("counter-irritation") or a distant site ("revulsion"), postulated from the theory that the patient's "system" could only sustain a fixed amount of inflammation and vascular excitement, are illusory.

Period Reference:

The Practice of Civil War Medicine and Surgery
The Elements of Materia Medica and Therapeutics – Jonathan Pereira, M.D. (Blanchard and Lee, Philadelphia, 1852) on the uses and administration of:
Strong Ammonia

Uses.– Ammonia is adapted for speedily rousing the action of the vascular and respiratory systems, and for the prompt alleviation of spasm. It is more especially fitted for fulfilling these indications when our object is at the same time to promote the action of the skin. It is calculated for states of debility with torpor or inactivity. It is also used. as an antacid and. local irritant.

1. *To produce local irritation, rubefaction, vesication, or destruction of the part.*– As a *local agent,* ammonia has been employed in a variety of diseases – some-times as a rubefacient or irritant, sometimes as a vesicant, and occasionally as a caustic. Thus it is employed as a rubefacient in rheumatic and neuralgic pains, and as a counter-irritant to relieve internal inflammations. As a local irritant, a weak solution has been injected into the vagina and uterus, to excite the catamenial discharge; but there are some objections to its use. Thus, it is a most unpleasant kind of remedy, especially to young females; moreover, the stoppage of this discharge is in many cases dependent on constitutional or remote causes, and, therefore, a topical remedy is not likely to be beneficial. Lavagna employed ten or fifteen drops of the solution, diluted with milk.

Sometimes ammonia is employed as a vesicatory; and it has two advantages over cantharides – a more speedy operation, and non-affection of the urinary organs. It may be employed either in the form of ointment or solution. As a caustic, the strong solution of ammonia may be sometimes used with advantage in the bites of rabid animals.

2. *The vapour of the solution of ammonia may be inhaled* when we wish to make a powerful impression on the nervous system – as in syncope, or to prevent an attack of epilepsy. To guard against or relieve fainting, ammoniacal inhalations are very powerful and useful: their instantaneous operation is frequently astonishing. Pinel says he

once saw an attack of epilepsy prevented by this means. The patient(a watchmaker) had intimations of the approaching paroxysm from certain feelings; but he found, by inhaling the vapour of ammonia, it was frequently prevented. In the case of a confirmed epilepsy, which I was in the habit of watching for some years, I think I have also seen analogous beneficial effects. I speak doubtfully, because it is so difficult to determine, in most cases, the actual approach of the fit. It is deserving of especial notice, that ammonia is useful in three conditions of the system, which, though produced by very different causes, present analogous symptoms; viz. idiopathic epilepsy – the insensibility and convulsions (? epilepsy) produced by loss of blood – and the insensibility and convulsions (? epilepsy) which poisonous doses of hydrocyanic acid give rise to. (See *ante,* p. 247; also *ammoniae sesquicarbonas.)* In asphyxia, ammoniacal inhalations have been strongly recommended by Sage, who says that he produced the apparent death of rabbits by immersion in water, and recovered them subsequently by the use of ammonia; and a case is mentioned of a man who had been submerged in the Seine for twenty minutes, and when taken out of the water, appeared lifeless, yet by the use of ammonia recovered; and a M. Routier, a surgeon of Amiens, is said to have restored a patient in the same way. That it may sometimes be of service I can readily believe, but it must be employed with great caution.

The employment of the vapour of ammonia, by Mr. Smee, as a topical expectorant, has been already noticed (see *ante,* p. 426).

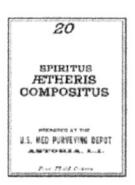

Spiritus Ætheris Compositus- (compound spirits of sulphuric ether, similar to Hoffman's Anodyne Liquor) - Colorless liquid

This is formally a stimulant, but its antispasmodic qualities are useful for treatment of nervous irritation causing sleeplessness and to prevent nausea and vomiting caused by other medications such as laudanum, without unwanted sedation. Perhaps the most frequent use is to treat the various milder symptoms of hysteria, including faintness, lowness of spirits, languor, palpitations, &etc. It is preferred over **Spiritus Ammoniæ Aromaticus** when the antispasmodic qualities are desired as indicated by the presence of palpiations, twitching, starting, &etc. The dose is one-half to two fludrachms in water, sweetened with sugar.

Modern Perspective:

Sulphuric ether alone - so called because it was produced by the action of sulphuric acid on alcohol, was used widely as an anesthetic. Union surgeons preferred chloroform due to a lesser explosive potential and less excitation of the patient during the initial introduction of the anesthetic (due to the greater potency of chloroform, which shortens this stage). Because of this effect, ether was classified as a "stimulant" with subsequent loss of consciousness being a "reaction".

This substance, with added alcohol and oil of wine, probably had no effect other than some sedation due jointly to the alcohol and the ether.

No specific "antispasmodic" effect - the effect imagined to combat any abrupt and recurring symptom, ranging from

abdominal cramps to neuralgic pains to epileptic seizures - would be expected.

The toxicity is that of alcohol.

Period Reference:

The Elements of Materia Medica and Therapeutics – Jonathan Pereira, M.D. (Blanchard and Lee, Philadelphia, 1852) on the uses and administration of:
Compound Spirits of Ether

1. **Medicinal Uses**. a. *Internal.–* Ether is principally valuable as a speedy and powerful agent in spasmodic and painful affections not dependent on local vascular excitement, and which are accompanied by a pale cold skin, and a small feeble pulse. If administered during a paroxysm of spasmodic asthma, it generally gives relief, but has no tendency to prevent the recurrence of attacks. In cramp of the stomach, singultus, and flatulent colic, its happy effects are well established. It is sometimes highly advantageous in a paroxysm of angina pectoris. During the passage of urinary or biliary calculi, it may be used as a substitute for, or in combination with, opium, to overcome the spasm of the ducts or tubes through which the calculus is passing. In the latter stages of continued fever, ether is sometimes admissible. It is employed to relieve the subsultus tendinum and hiccup. Desbois de Rochefort administered it in intermittent fevers. He gave it about half an hour before the expected paroxysm; it acted as a mild diaphoretic, and prevented the recurrence of the attack. Headache of the kind popularly called nervous, that is, unconnected with vascular excitement, is sometimes speedily relieved by ether. I have found it beneficial principally in females of delicate habits. In such it occasionally gives itnmediate relief, even when the throbbing of the temporal vessels and suffusion of the eyes (symptoms which usually contraindicate the employment of ether) would seem to show the existence of excitement of the cerebral vessels.

In flatulence of the stomach it may be taken in combination with some aromatic water. Against sea-sickness it should be swallowed in a glass of white wine. Durande recommends a mixture of three parts ether, and two oil of turpentine, as a solvent for biliary calculi. Bourdier employed ether to expel tape-worm. He administered it, by the stomach and rectum, in an infusion of male fern, giving a dose of castor-oil an hour after. In faintness and lowness of spirits, it is a popular remedy. In poisoning by hemlock and mushrooms, it has been employed. In asphyxia it has been used with benefit.

The vapour of ether is inhaled in spasmodic asthma, chronic catarrh, and dyspnoea, hooping-cough, and to relieve the effects caused by the accidental inhalation of chlorine gas. It may be used by dropping some ether in hot water, and inspiring the vapour mixed with steam; or it may be dropped on sugar, which is to be held in the mouth. The inhalation of the vapour of the ethereal tincture of hemlock is occasionally useful in relieving spasmodic affections of the respiratory organs, and has been recommended in phthisical cases.

b . External – The principal external use of ether is to produce cold by its speedy evaporation. Thus, in strangulated hernia, it, may be dropped on the tumour and allowed. to evaporate freely: by this means, a considerable degree of cold is produced, and, in consequence, the bulk of the part diminished, whereby the reduction of the hernia is facilitated. Dropped on the forehead, or applied by means of a piece of thin muslin, ether diminishes vascular excitement, by the cold produced from its evaporation, and. Is exceedingly efficacious in headache and inflammatory conditions of the brain. In burns and scalds, it may also be employed as a refrigerant. If its evaporation be stopped or checked, as by covering it with a compress, it acts as a local irritant, causing rubefaction, and, by long-continued application, vesication. It is used with friction as a local stimulant.

2. **Pharmaceutical Uses.**– Ether is employed. in the preparation of the Compound Spirit of Sulphuric Ether. Ether, or its alcoholic solution, is also used to extract the active principles of certain drugs, as of Lobelia, Aloes, Musk, &c. The solutions are called Ethereal Tinctures *(Tincturae Ethereae),* or by the French pharmacologists

E*theroles*. These may be, conveniently prepared by percolation. Ether is of assistance in determining the purity of some medicinal substances, as of Aconitina and Veratria, which are very soluble in it. It is employed in toxicological researches to remove Bichloride of Mercury from organic mixtures. [A solution of gun-cotton or xyloidine in ether is well known and extensively employed in pharmacy under the name of *Collodion*– Ed.]

Administration.– It may be given in doses of from one-half to two drachm, a teaspoonful is the ordinary quantity. This dose may be repeated at short intervals. It is usually exhibited in some aromatic water, and frequently in combination with other antispasmodics and stimulants, as ammonia or valerian. "It may be perfectly incorporated. with water, or any aqueous mixture, by rubbing it up with spermaceti, employed in the proportion of two grains for each fluidrachm of the ether.'"

Antidotes.– In cases of poisoning by ether, the same treatment is to be adopted as before recommended in cases of poisoning by alcohol.

SPIRITUS AETHERIS COMPOSITUS; *Compound Sirit of Sulphuric Ether* - This preparation is commonly called *Hoffmann's Mineral Anodyne Liquor*; being made in imitation of a preparation described by Hoffmann, which it is said he was taught by an apothecary of the dame of Martmeier. This preparation is sometimes employed as an adjunct to laudanum, to prevent the nausea which the latter excites in certain habits. Its dose is from one-half to two drachm in any proper vehicle.

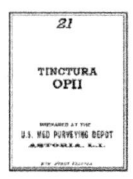

Tinctura Opii (tincture of opium; laudanum) - Reddish-brown liquid

Opium may best be characterized as a stimulant narcotic; the main use is for pain relief (anodyne). The dose is variable, 10 minums to a fluid ounce until the effect is achieved. This form is preferred over solid opium when an immediate effect is desired.

Modern Perspective:

Opium effectively relieves pain and checks diarrhea (causing constipation with chronic use). Opium in its various forms represented the only effective pain reliever available to the civil war surgeon short of anesthesia. Morphine is still the gold standard for pain relief.

The civil war surgeon was hampered by the lack of an effective pain reliever for lesser pain. Aspirin was not widely available until the turn of the century for pain and fever relief, although folk remedies using bark preparations containing salicylates (related to aspirin) dated back to Native American use.

Period Reference:

The Elements of Materia Medica and Therapeutics – Jonathan Pereira, M.D. (Blanchard and Lee, Philadelphia, 1852) on the uses and administration of:
Opium

Uses.– Opium is undoubtedly the most important and valuable remedy of the whole Materia Medica. For other medicines we have one or more substitutes; but for opium none, at least in the large majority of cases in which its peculiar and beneficial influence is required. Its good effects are not, as is the case with some valuable medicines, remote and contingent, but they are immediate, direct, and obvious; and its operation is not attended with pain or discomfort. Farthermore, it is applied, and with the greatest success, to the relief of maladies of every day's occurrence, some of which are attended with the most acute human suffering- These circumstances, with others not necessary here to enumerate, conspire to give to opium an interest not possessed by any other article of the Materia Medica.

We employ it to fulfil various indications; some of which have been already noticed. Thus we exhibit it, under certain regulations, to rnitigate pain, to allay spasm, to promote sleep, to relieve nervous restlessness, to produce perspiration and to check profuse mucous discharges from the bronchial tubes and gastro-intes- tinal canal. But experience has proved its value in relieving some diseases in which not one of these indications can be at all times distinctly traced.

1. *In Fevers.–* The consideration of the use of opium in fever presents peculiar difficulties. Though certain symptoms which occur in the course of this disease are, under some circumstances, most advantageously treated by opium, *yet, with* one or more of these symptoms present, opium may, notwithstanding, be a very inappropriate remedy. The propriety or impropriety of its use, in such cases, must be determined by other circumstances, which, however, are exceedingly difficult to define and characterize. It should always be employed with great caution, giving it in small doses, and carefully watching its effects. The symptoms for which it has been resorted to are, *watchfulness, great restlessness, delirium, tremor,* and *diarrhea.* When watchfulness and great restlessness are disproportionate, from first to last, to the disorder of the vascular system, or of the constitution at large; or when these symptoms continue after excitement of the vascular system has been subdued by appropriate depletives, opium frequently proves a highly valuable remedy; nay,

the safety of the patient often arises from its judicious employment. The same remarks also apply to the employment of opium for the relief of delirium; but it may be added that, in patients who have been addicted to the use of spirituous liquors, the efficacy of opium in allaying delirium is greatest. Yet I have seen opium fail to relieve the delirium of fever, even when given apparently under favourable circumstances; and I have known opium restore the consciousness of a delirious patient, and yet the case has terminated fatally. If the skin be damp, and the tongue moist, it rarely, I think, proves injurious. The absence, however, of these favourable conditions by no means precludes the employment of opium; but its efficacy is more doubtful. Dr. Holland suggests that the condition of the pupil may serve as a guide in some doubtful cases; where it is contracted, opium being contraindicated. A similar suggestion with respect to the use of belladonna was made by Dr. Graves, to which I have offered some objections. When sopor or coma supervenes in fever, the use of opium generally proves injurious. Recently, the combination of opium and emetic tartar has been strongly recommended in fever with much cerebral disturbance, by Dr. Law and Dr. Graves.

2. In Inflammatory Diseases.– Opium has long been regarded as an objectionable remedy in inflammation; but it is one we frequently resort to, either for the purpose of palliating particular symptoms, or even as a powerful auxiliary antiphlogistic remedy. The statement of Dr. Young, " that opium was improper in all those diseases in which bleeding was necessary," is, therefore, by no means correct in a very considerable number of instances. The objects for which opium is usually exhibited in inflammatory diseases are to mitigate excessive pain, to allay spasm, to relieve great restlessness, to check excessive secretion, and to act as an antiphlogistic. In employing it as an anodyne, we are to bear in mind that it is applicable to those cases only in which the pain is disproportionate to the local vascular excitement; and even then it must be employed with considerable caution; for to "stupefy the sensibility to pain, or to suspend any particular disorder of function, unless we can simultaneously lessen or remove the causes which create it, is often but to interpose a veil between our judgment and the impending danger." As an antiphlogistic, it is best given in conjunction with calomel, as recommended by Dr. R. Hamilton, of Lynn. The practice, however, does not prove equally successful in all forms of inflammation. It is best adapted for the disease when it affects membranous parts," and is much less beneficial in inflammation of the parenchymatous structure of organs. In *gastritis* and *enteritis* the use of opium has been strongly recommended by the late Dr. Armstrong. After bleeding the patient to syncope, a full opiate (as 80 or 100 drops of the tincture, or three grains of soft opium) is to be administered; and if the stomach reject it, we may give it by injection. It acts on the skin, induces quiet and refreshing sleep, and prevents what is called the hemorrhagic reaction. If the urgent symptoms return when the patient awakes, the same mode of treatment is to be followed, but combining calomel with the opium. A. third venesection is seldom required. In *peritonitis,* the same plan of treatment is to be adopted; but warm, moist applications are on no account to be omitted. Of the great value of opiates in *puerperal fever,* 'abundant evidence has been adduced by Dr. Ferguson. In *cystitis,* opium, preceded "and accompanied by bloodletting and the warm bath, is a valuable remedy; it relieves the scalding pain, by diminishing the sensibility of this viscus to the presence of the urine, and also counteracts the spasmodic contractions. In *inflammation of the walls of the pelvis of the kidney, and also of the ureters,* especially when brought on by the presence of a calculus, opium is a most valuable remedy; it diminishes the sensibility of these parts, and prevents spasm; farthermore, it relaxes the ureters, and thereby facilitates the passage of the calculus. in *inflammat,ion of the gall-ducts,* produced by calculus, opium is likewise serviceable; but, as in the last-mentioned case, bloodletting and the warm bath should be employed simultaneously with it. In *inflammation of the mucous membranes,* attended with increased secretion, opium is a most valuable remedy. Thus, in *pulmonary catarrh,* when the first stage of the disease has passed by, and the mucous secretion is fully established, opium is frequently very beneficial; it diminishes the sensibility of the bronchial membrane to cold air, and thereby prevents cough. In severe forms of the disease, blood-letting ought to be premised. Given at the commencement of the disease, Dr. Holland says that twenty or thirty drops of laudanum will often arrest it altogether. In *diarrhea,* opium, in mild cases, is often sufficient of itself to cure the disease; it diminishes the increased muscular contractions and increased sensibility (thereby relieving pain), and at the same time checks excessive secretion. Aromatics and. chalk are advantageously combined with it. In violent cases, blood-letting should precede or accompany it. *Mild* or *English cholera,* the disease which has been so long known in this country, and which consists in irritation or inflammation of the mucous lining of the stomach, is generally most successfully treated by the use of opium; two or three doses will, in slight cases, be sufficient to effect a cure. When opium fails, the hydrocyanic acid is occasionally most effective. In *dysentery,* opium has been found very serviceable; it is best given in combination with either ipecacuanha or calomel. I have already stated that, in *inflammation, of the parenchymatous tissues of organs,* the use of opium is less frequently beneficial, but often injurious. Thus, in *inflammation of the cerebral substance,* it is highly objectionable, since it increases the determination of blood to the head, and disposes to coma. In *peripneumonia,* it is for the most part injurious; partly by its increasing the febrile symptoms, partly by its diminishing the bronchial secretion, and probably, also, by retarding the arterialization of the blood, and thereby increasing the general disorder of system. It must be admitted, however, that there are circumstances under which its use, in this disease, is justifiable. Thus, in acute peripneumonia, when bloodletting has been carried as far as the safety of the patient will admit, but without the subsidence of the disease, I have seen the repeated use of opium and calomel of essential service. Again, in the advanced stages of pneumonic inflammation, when the difficulty of breathing has abated, opium is sometimes beneficially employed to allay painful cough, and produce sleep. In *inflammation of the substance of the Liver,* opium is seldom beneficial; it checks the excretion, if not the secretion, of bile, and increases costiveness. In *rheumatic,* opium frequently evinces its happiest effects. In acute forms of the disease it is given in combination with calomel, as recommended by Dr. R. Hamilton – bloodletting being usually premised. From half a grain to two grains of opium should be given at a dose. Dr. Hope recommends gr. 7 or gr. 10 of calomel to be combined with each dose of opium. It is not necessary, or even proper, in ordinary cases, to affect the mouth by the calomel; though to this statement exceptions exist. The use of mercury may even, in some cases, be objectionable; and in such, Dover's powder will be found the best form of exhibition. This plan of treatment is well adapted for the diffuse or fibrous form of acute rheumatism; but it does not prove equally successful in the synovial forms of the disease. It is also valuable in chronic rheumatism.

8. *In Diseases of the Brain and Spinal Cord.–* In some cerebro-spinal diseases great benefit arises from the use of opium; while in other cases injury only can result from its employment. The latter effect is to be expected in inflammation of the brain, and in apoplectic cases. In other words, in those cerebral maladies obviously connected with, or dependent on, an excited condition of the vascular system of the brain, opium acts injuriously. Rut there are many disordered conditions of the cerebro-spinal functions, the intensity of which bears no proportion to that of the derangement of the vascular system of the brain; and there are other deviations from the healthy functions in which no change in the cerebral circulation can be detected. In these cases, opium or morphia frequently evinces its best effects. In *insanity,* its value has been properly insisted on by Dr. Seymour. He, as well as Messrs. Reverley and Phillips, employed the acetate of morphia. Its good effects were manifested rather in the low, desponding, or melancholic forms of the disease, than in the excited conditions; though I have seen great relief obtained in the latter form of the disease by full doses. Opium is sometimes employed by drunkards to relieve *intoxication..* I knew a medical man addicted to drinking, and who, for many years, was accustomed to take a large dose of laudanum whenever he was intoxicated. and was called to see a patient. On one occasion, being more than ordinarily inebriated, he swallowed an excessive dose of laudanum, and died in a few hours of apoplexy.

In *delirium tremens,* the efficacy of opium is almost universally admitted. Its effects, however, require to be carefully watched; for large doses of it, frequently repeated; sometimes hasten coma and other bad symptoms. If there be much fever, or evident marks of determination of blood to the head, it should be used with great caution, and ought to be preceded by loss of blood, cold applications to the head, and other antiphlogistic measures. Though opium is to be looked on as a chief remedy in this disease, yet it is not to be regarded as a specific. Dr. Law speaks in high terms of its association with emetic tartar. I have before noticed the use of opium in alleviating some of the *cerebral symptoms which occur during fever.*

In *spasmodic and convulsive diseases* opium is a most important remedy. In *local spasms produced by topical irritants,* it is a most valuable agent, as I have already stated; for example, *in spasm of the gall-ducts* or *of the ureters,* brought on by the presence of calculi; in colic, and in *painful spasmodic contractions of the bladder,* or *rectum,* or *uterus.* In *spasmodic stricture* opium is sometimes useful. In genuine *spasmodic asthma,* which probably depends on a spasmodic condition of the muscular fibres investing the bronchial tubes, a full dose of opium generally gives temporary relief; but the recurrence of the paroxysms is seldom influenced by opium. There are several reasons for believing that one effect of narcotics in dyspnea is to diminish the necessity for respiration. Laennec states that when given to relieve the extreme dyspnea of mucous catarrh, it frequently produces a speedy but temporary cessation of the disease; and if we explore the respiration by the stethoscope, we find it the same as during the paroxysm – a proof that the benefit obtained consists simply in a diminution of the necessity for respiration. That the necessities of the system for atmospheric air vary at different periods, and from different circumstances, is sufficiently established by the experiments of Dr. Prout, and it appears that they are diminished during sleep, at which time, according to Dr. Edwards, the transpiration is increased. Moreover, the phenomena of hibernating animals also bear on this point; for during their state of torpidity, or hibernation, their respiration is proportionally diminished.

In the *convulsive diseases (chorea, epilepsy,* and *tetanus)* opium has been used, with variable success; in fact, the conditions of system under which these affections occur, may be, at different times, of an opposite nature; so that a remedy which is proper in one case is often improper in another. In *tetanus,* opium was at one time a favourite remedy, and is undoubtedly at times a remedy of considerable value. But it is remarkable that the susceptibility of the system to its influence is greatly diminished during tetanus. I have already referred to the enormous quantities which may, at this time, be taken with impunity. In 128 cases noticed by Mr. Curling, opium in various forms, and in conjunction with other remedies, was employed in 84 cases; and of these, 45 recovered. Notwithstanding, however, the confidence of the profession in its efficacy is greatly diminished.

Lastly, opium occasionally proves serviceable in several forms of *headache,* especially after loss of blood. I have seen it give great relief in some cases of what are commonly termed nervous headaches; while in others, with apparently the same indications, it has proved injurious. Chomel applied, with good effect, opium cerate to a blistered surface of the scalp, to relieve headache.

4. *In Diseases of the Chest.–* In some affections of the heart and of the organs of respiration opium is beneficial. I have already alluded to its employment in *catarrh, peripnenmonia,* and *spasmodic asthma.* In the first of these maladies caution is often requisite in its use. "In an aged person, for example, suffering under *chronic bronchitis* or *catarrhal influenza* – and gasping, it may be, under the difficulties of cough and expectoration – an opiate, by suspending these very struggles, may become the cause of danger and death. The effort here is needed for the recovery of free respiration; and if suppressed too long, mucus accumulates in the bronchial cells, its extrication thence becomes impossible, and breathing ceases altogether."

5. *In Maladies of the Digestive Organs* – I have already referred to the use of opium in *gastritis, enteritis, peritonitis, diarrhea, dysentery, colic, the passage of gall-stones,* and in *hepatitis.* With respect to the use of opium *in hepatic affections,* I am disposed to think, with Dr. Holland, that, with the exception of the painful passage of a gall-stone through the ducts, there is scarcely a complaint of the liver and its appendages "where opium may not be said to be

hurtful, though occasionally and indirectly useful when combined with other.means." *In poisoning by acrid substances* opium is used with advantage to lessen the susceptibility of the alimentary canal, and thereby to diminish the violence of the operation of these local irritants. Cantharides, all the drastic purgatives, when taken in excessive doses (as elaterium, colocynth, gamboge, scamrnony, and craton oil or seeds), and Arum *maculatum,* may be mentioned as examples of the substances alluded to. Besides the above-mentioned beneficial operation, opium allays the spasmodic contractions of *the* bowels, relieves pain, and checks inordinate secretion and exhalation.

In poisoning by corrosives (the strong mineral acids and alkalies, for example), opium diminishes the sensibility of the alimentary canal; it cannot, of course, alter the chemical influence of the poisons, but it may prove useful by allaying the consequences of inflammation.

As meconic acid is said to be an antidote in cases of poisoning by corrosive sublimate, opium, in full doses, may perhaps be administered with some advantage when other antidotes cannot be procured.

In poisoning by the preparations of arsenic, of lead, and of copper, opium is sometimes found useful.

6. *In maladies of the urino-genital apparatus* opium is a most valuable remedy. It mitigates pain, allays spasmodic action, checks copious mucous secretion, and diminishes irritation. Its use for one or more of these purposes in *nephritis, cystitis, the passage of urinary calculi,* and *spasmodic stricture,* has been already pointed *out. In irritable bladder* it is an invaluable remedy, especially in conjunction with liquor potassae. *In irritation* and *various painful affections of the uterus,* and in *chordee,* the value of opium is well known. In the treatment of the *phosphatic diathesis* it is the only remedy that can be employed, according to Dr. Prout, to diminish the unnatural irritability of the system.

Of all remedies for that hitherto intractable malady, *diabetes,* opium has been found to give the most relief. Under its use the specific gravity, saccharine quality, and quantity of urine have been diminished. It has not, however, hitherto succeeded in permanently curing this disease. Dr. Prout has also found it serviceable when there is an excess *of urea in the urine.*

7. *As an Anodyne.–* To relieve pain by dulling the sensibility of the body, opium is, of all substances, the most useful, and the most to be relied on for internal exhibition. We sometimes use it to alleviate the pain of inflammation, as already mentioned; to diminish spasm and the sensibility of the part in calculi of the gall-ducts, in the ureters, and even when in the urinary bladder; to relieve pain in the various forms of scirrhus and carcinoma, in which diseases opium is our sheet-anchor; to allay the pain arising from the presence of foreign bodies in wounds; to prevent or relieve after-pains; to diminish the pain of menstruation; and, lastly, as an anodyne in neuralgia. As a *benember* or *topical anodyne* it is greatly inferior to aconite. Hence, in neuralgia, the latter is much more successful than opium. (See *Aconitum.)*

8. *In Hemorrhages.–* Opium is at times serviceable to obviate certain *ill effects of hemorrhages;* as when there is great irritability attended with a small and frequent pulse, and also to relieve that painful throbbing about the head so often observed after large evacuations of blood. In or immediately after *uterine hemorrhage* the use of opium has been objected to, on the ground that it might prevent the contraction of the womb; but where the employment of opium is otherwise indicated, this theoretical objection deserved no weight. In *bronchial hemorrhage* it is at times a valuable remedy, and may be associated with acetate of lead (notwithstanding the chemical objections to the mixture) with good effect.

9. *In Mortification.–* When mortification is attended with excessive pain, opium is resorted to. In that kind of mortification called *gangrene senilis,* which commences without any visible cause, by a small purple spot on the toes, heels, or other parts of the extremities, and which sometimes arises from an ossified condition of the arteries, Mr. Pott strongly recommended opium, in conjunction with a stimulating plan of treatment, and experience has fully proved its great efficacy.

10. *In Venereal Diseases.—* Opium is frequently employed in venereal diseases to prevent the action of mercurials on the bowels during salivation; also to allay the pain of certain venereal sores, and venereal diseases of the bones. By some it has, in addition, been employed as an anti-venereal remedy; and, according to Michaelis and others, with success. Moreover, it is stated by Dr. Ananian, who practised at Constantinople, that those persons who were in the habit of taking opium rarely contracted the venereal disease. But opium possesses no specific anti-venereal powers. It has appeared to me, on several occasions, to promote the healing of venereal sores.

11. In various forms of *ulcers,* and in *granulating wounds* the efficacy of opium has been satisfactorily established by Mr. Skey. Richter and others had already noticed its good effects; but their statements had attracted little attention. Mr. Grant, in 1785, pointed out the efficacy of opium in the treatment of foul ulcers, attended with a bad discharge, and much pain. He ascribed these symptoms to "morbid irritability," which the opium removed. Its use is prejudicial in ulcers attended with inflammation, in the florid or sanguineous temperament, and in childhood. But in the chronic or callous ulcer, in the so-called varicose ulcer, in recent ulcers (from wounds), in which granulation proceeds slowly, or in other cases, the efficacy of opium, administered in small doses (as ten drops of laudanum three times daily), is most manifest, especially in elderly persons, and in those whose constitutions have been debilitated by disease, labour, spirituous liquors, &c. It appears to promote the most genial warmth, to give energy to the extreme arteries, and thereby to maintain an equal balance of the circulation throughout every part of the body, and to animate the dormant energies of healthy action.

12. The *external application* of opium is comparatively but little resorted to, and for two reasons: in the first place, its topical effects are slight; and secondly, its specific effects on the brain and general system are not readily produced through the skin. Aconite and belladonna greatly exceed opium in their topical effects. The following are some of the local uses of opium: In *ophthalmia,* the wine of opium is dropped into the eye when there is excessive pain

(see *Vinum Opia*). In *painful and foul sores,* opiates are used with occasional good effects. Mr. Grant applied the tincture twice a day, in an oatmeal poultice, to irritable sores. Opiate *frictions* have been employed as topical anodynes, and to affect. the general system. - Thus, in *chronic rheumatism and sprains,* the opium liniment proves a useful application. In *maniacal delirium,* as well as some other cerebral disorders, Mr. Ward employed, with apparently beneficial effects, opiate frictions; for example, one-half ounce of opium, mixed with gr. 4 of camphor, 4 scruples of lard, and one drachm of olive oil. In *neuralgic affections,* an opiate cerate, or finely powdered hydrochlorate of morphia, applied to a blistered surface, occasionally gives relief. In *gastrodynia,* it may be applied in the same way to the epigastrium (Holland). In *gonorrhea and gleet,* opium injections have been used. In *spasmodic stricture, diseases of the prostate gland,* and in g*onorrhoea to prevent chordee,* an opiate suppository is a useful form of employing opium, especially where it is apt to disagree with the stomach. In *nervous and spasmodic affections* (as some forms of asthma), the endermic application of opium or morphia, applied along the course of the spine, is often singularly beneficial, when all methods of depletion and counter-irritation have proved utterly unavailing (Holland). In *toothache,* opium is applied to the hollow of a carious tooth. Dr. Row speaks in the highest terms of the efficacy of the external application of opium *in inflammatory diseases,* but especially *bronchitis* and *croup.*

Administration.– Opium is given, *in substance,* in the form of pill, powder, lozenge, or electuary. The dose is subject to great variation, depending on the age and habits of the patient, the nature of the disease, and the particular object for which we wish to employ it. In a general way, we consider from an eighth of a grain to half a grain a *small dose* for an adult. We give it to this extent in persons unaccustomed to its use, when we require its stimulant effects, and in mild catarrhs and diarrhoeas. From half a grain to two grains we term a *medium dose,* and employ it in this quantity as an ordinary anodyne and soporific. From two to five grains we denominate a *full* or *large dose,* and give it to relieve excessive pain, violent spasm, in some inflammatory diseases after bloodletting, in tetanus, &c. These are by no means to be regarded as the limits of the use of opium. *Opium pills (pilulae opii)* may be prepared either with crude or powdered opium. The latter has the advantage of a more speedy operation, in consequence of its more ready solution in the gastric liquor. Employed as a *suppository,* opium is used in larger doses than when given by the stomach. Five grains, made into a cylindric mass with soap, may be introduced into the rectum, to allay irritation in the urinogenital organs.

Bruce A. Evans, M.D.

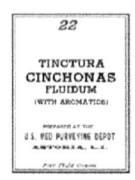

Tinctura Cinchonas Fluidum (with aromatics) - Reddish-yellow liquid

(Documented in use by Indians prior to Spanish invasion in 16th Century)

This medicine is an alcohol-based preparation of cinchona bark. It has the same effects on the system as the constituent quinine, but at one-third the strength. It is much more irritating to the stomach and bowels, and is therefore usually used in small doses as a tonic, or as an adjunct to the quinine salt for fever. As a tonic, tincture of chinchona causes increased appetite, promotes digestion, increases the force of the pulse, promotes the process of nutrition, and generally stimulates vital processes. It is easier of the stomach than decoctions of the bark and less bitter, and is also therefore useful in simple dyspepsia, although probably not superior to simple bitters for this use. It is particularly useful in general debility, or debility due to chronic suppurative disease. For fever it is used with quinine, especially when the stimulant effect of the alcohol is desired in low or putrid fevers. As a specific for intermittent fever without a typhoid or low fever taint, the quinine salt preparation is superior and better tolerated in the high doses often required.

The dose is 1 to 4 fluidrachms, two to four times per day in chronic debility or low fever, and with each quinine dose in intermittent fever.

Modern Perspective:

This is one of the few specific and effective remedies available in these times when used for the appropriate indication. The active ingredient of cinchona – quinine – is an effective treatment of malaria ("intermittent fever" as called during this time). In the early to mid-19th century, it was recognized that a disease charactered by severe bouts of fever and delirium ending in drenching seats, occurring at very regular and therefore predictable intervals with no fever in between could be effectively treated with preparations of chinchona bark.

The bark was therefore felt to be an effective treatment for febrile disease in general, although it was observed soon enough that patients with other fever patterns such as "continued fever" (steady or mildly fluctuating), "hectic fever" (swinging irregularly and wildly to high temperatures), or "remittent fever" (periodic but not returning to normal between it's not so regular and predictable attacks) did not in fact respond. We know now that quinine directly attacks the blood cell parasite that causes malaria ("intermittent fever") but does not have a generalized effect on the other diseases causing the above noted fever patterns, and does not have a general fever-lowering effect as do aspirin, ibuprofen, and other similar more modern anti-inflammatory drugs.

The "halo effect" from the drug's success probably led to its use in smaller doses of this preparation as a general "tonic". This use lasted well into this century as the popular carbonated quinine flavored drinks attest.

Quinine can be quite toxic to the central nervous system and the heart, but this preparation is so much weaker in quinine content that toxicity was likely not a problem.

From a modern perspective then, this was an effective medication in the treatment of true intermittent fever - ague or malaria - but ineffective in general febrile disease.

Period Reference:

The Elements of Materia Medica and Therapeutics – Jonathan Pereira, M.D. (Blanchard and Lee, Philadelphia, 1852) on the uses and administration of:

Uses.– From the preceding account of the physiological effects of cinchona, some of the indications and contra-indications for its use may be readily inferred thus its topical employment is obviously indicated in cases of local relaxation, with or without excessive secretion; also in poisoning by those agents whose compounds with tannic acid are difficultly soluble, and, therefore, not readily absorbed. But as a topical remedy, or astringent, cinchona is greatly inferior to many other agents which contain a much larger quantity of tannic acid. The contra-indications for the local use of cinchona, are, states of irritation (nervous or vascular), and. of inflammation. In these conditions it aggravates the morbid symptoms.

The indications for its use, as a general or constitutional remedy, are, debility with atony and laxity of the solids, and profuse discharges from the secreting organs. I have observed that it proves less successful, and often quite fails, when the complexion is chlorotic or anaemic; in such cases chalybeates often succeed where cinchona is useless or injurious. As contra-indications for its employment, may be enumerated acute inflammation, inflammatory fever, plethora, active hemorrhages, inflammatory dropsies, &c. To these may be added, an extremely debilitated condition of the digestive and assimilative organs. Thus, patients recovering from protracted fever are at first unable to support the use of bark, which acts as an irritant to the stomach, and causes an increase of the febrile symptoms. In such cases I have found infusion of calumba a good preparative for cinchona.

Hitherto, I have referred to those indications only which have an obvious relation to the known physiological effects of cinchona. But the diseases in which this remedy manifests the greatest therapeutic power, are those which assume an intermittent or periodical type. Now, in such, the *methodus medeni* is quite inexplicable; and, therefore, the remedy has been called a *specific,* an *antiperiodic,* and a *febrifuge.* But the more intimately we become acquainted with the pathology of disease, and the operation of medicines, the less evidence have we of the specific influence of particular medicines over particular maladies. Some diseases, however, are exceedingly obscure; their seat or nature, and the condition of system under which they occur, or the cause of their occurrence, being little known. There are also many medicines, the precise action of which is imperfectly understood, but which evidently exercise a most important, though to us quite inexplicable, influence over the system. Now, it sometimes happens that imperfectly known diseases are most remarkably influenced by remedies, the agency of which we cannot comprehend; in other words, we can trace no known relation between the physiological effects of the remedy and its therapeutical influence. This incomprehensible relationship exists between arsenic and lepra; between the cinchona bark and ague. But though this connection is to us mysterious (for I do not admit the various hypotheses which have been formed to account for it), we are not to conclude that it is necessarily more intimate than that which exists in ordinary cases.

1. *In periodical or intermittent, diseases.*– The system is subject to several diseases, which assume a *periodical* form; that is, they disappear and return at regular intervals. When the patient appears to be quite well during the interval (i.e. when the intermission is perfect and regular) the disease is called an *intermittent,;* whereas it is called *remittent* when the second paroxysm makes its appearance before the first has wholly subsided (i.e. when the disease presents exacerbations and remissions, but not intermissions). The pathology of these

affections is involved in great obscurity, and the cause or causes of their periodicity are completely unknown. Various circumstances, however, induce us to regard intermittent maladies as morbid affections of the nervous system; for the phenomena of periodicity, both healthy and morbid, seem to be essentially nervous. One of the most curious circumstances connected with the history of these diseases is the facility with which they are sometimes cured. It is well known that sudden and powerful impressions, both mental and corporeal (as those caused by terror, alcohol, opium, cinchona, arsenious acid, &c.), made during the intermission, will sometimes prevent the return of the succeeding paroxysm; and occasionally from that time all morbid phenomena disappear. In remittent diseases, on the other hand, the same impressions are much less frequently successful, and sometimes, instead of palliating, exasperate the symptoms. The agents which are capable, under certain circumstances, of making these curative impressions, are apparently so dissimilar in their nature and physiological action, that we can trace in their *methodus medendi* scarcely anything in common, save that of making a powerful impression on the nervous system. Of these *anti-periodic* agents, cinchona and arsenious acids stands pre-eminent for their greater frequency of success, and, therefore, are those usually resorted to. I have already (see p. 685) made some remarks on their relative therapeutical value. They differ in two particulars; First, cinchona may be given, as an antiperiodic, in any quantity which the stomach can bear; whereas, arsenious acid must be exhibited in cautiously-regulated doses; secondly, there are two modes of attempting the cure of an intermittent by cinchona; one is, to put an immediate stop to the disease by the use of very large doses of the remedy given a few hours prior to the recurrence of the paroxysm – the other is, to distinguish the disease gradually by the exhibition of moderate doses at short intervals during the whole period of the intermission, so that the violence of every succeeding paroxysm is somewhat less than that of the preceding one; but in the case of arsenious acid, the latter method is alone safe, and, therefore, to be adopted.

It has been asserted that cinchona is admissible in the interval only of an intermittent fever; and that, if it be exhibited during the paroxysm, it has a tendency to prevent the subsidence of the latter. But this statement is much overcharged. Morton and others have given it in almost every stage without injury. Dr. Heberden observes, "the only harm which I believe would follow from taking the bark, even in the middle of the fit is, that it might occasion a sickness, and might harass the patient by being vomited up, and might set him against it." It is, however, more efficacious during, the interval, though it may not be absolutely hurtful in the paroxysm. Dr. Cullen was strongly of opinion that the nearer the exhibition of the cinchona is to the time of accession, the more certainly effectual will it be. I have already stated (vol. i. p. 685) that arsenious acid may be given with good effect during the whole period (paroxysm and intermission) of the disease.

A very necessary condition to its perfect success is that it sit well on the stomach; for if it occasion vomiting or purging, it is much less likely to act beneficially. Hence an emetic and a purgative are recommended to precede its employment. The use of these is more especially necessary if the disease be recent. For an adult, about fifteen grains of ipecacuanha, with a grain of tartarized antimony, may be exhibited as an emetic, unless there be symptoms of determination to the brain, or of inflammation of the digestive organs. A senna draught, with a calomel pill, forms a good purgative. To enable it to sit well on the stomach, cinchona (or the

sulphate of quina) is frequently given in conjunction with aromatics. The infusion or decoction of cinchona, though much less effective, is, however, less liable to disturb the stomach than the powder of cinchona or the sulphate of quinn. Opium is sometimes a necessary adjunct to cinchona to prevent its runuing oR' by the bowels. In some cases where the stomach was too irritable to admit of the administration of cinchona or sulphate of quina by the *mouth,* these agents have been otherwise introduced into the system. Thus, *clyster* of cinchona were used by Helvetius, Torti, and Baglivi. Van Swieten says he has often seen this method successful in infants, but that it takes three times as much bark as would suffice if the remedy were swallowed. *Cataplasms* of cinchona have also been employed. Rosenstein applied them to the abdomen, Torti to the wrist. Alexander cured an ague by a *pediluvium* of decoction of cinchona, but Heberden tried it without success. *Bark jackets* were employed with success in the agues of children, by Dr.Pye. They consisted of waistcoats between whose layers powdered cinchona was quilted. The *dry* powder of cinchona has been *applied to the skin;* thus, Dr. Darwin strewed it in the patient's bed. Chrestien successfully used the tincture and alcoholic extract by the *intraleptic method.* More recently, sulphate of quina has been employed in the same way. The last-mentioned operation has also been applied by the *endermic method,* but this mode of using it is sometimes attended with intense pain and an eschar. To infants at the breast, Rosenstein advises its indirect exhibition *by the nurse,* in whose milk its active principle is administered to the child. More recently, sulphate of quina mixed with tobacco (in the proportion of fifteen grains of the former to an ounce of the latter) has been employed as a *snuff* in intermittent headache.

Cinchona and its preparations prove most successful in the simple or uncomplicated form of intermittent; that is, where the disease appears to be purely nervous. But when agues are accompanied with inflammatory excitement or with visceral disease, cinchona generally proves either useless or injurious. In remittents it proves much less successful than in regularly-formed intermittents. In all these cases we endeavour to promote the efficiency of the cinchona by reducing the disease to the form of a pure or simple intermittent. The means to effect this must of course depend on a variety of circumstances; but bloodletting, both general and local, purgatives, and diaphoretics, are those which for the most part will be found. available. Under some circumstances, mercury given in alterative doses, or even *as* a very slight sialogogue, proves beneficial.

Intermittent fevers are not the only periodical diseases in which cinchona has been found beneficial. It is a remedy which has proved serviceable in several other cases in which a paroxysm (of pain, spasm, inflammation, hemorrhage, or fever) returns at stated periods. Thus, intermittent neuralgia, rheumatism, headache, amaurosis, catarrh, ophthalmia, stricture, &c. have been greatly benefited by its use. Some of these affections have been regarded as *masked agues.* When periodical diseases recur at uncertain periods, as in the case of epilepsy, no particular advantage can be expected from the use of cinchona.

2• *In continued fever.* – In the latter stage of continued fever, when the vital powers are beginning to sink, and when there is no marked and decided symptom of inflammatory disease of the brain or digestive organs, cinchona or sulphate of quina sometimes proves highly beneficial. If the tongue be dry, as well as furred, and the skin hot and dry, no advantage, but the reverse, can be anticipated from its employment. It is most applicable to the low forms of fever occurring in debilitated constitutions. When exacerbations or remissions, however indistinct, occur at regular periods, the administration of cinchona is the more likely to be followed

by good effects. Under the preceding circumstances there can scarcely be two opinions as to the admissibility of bark. But on the general propriety of administering this remedy in continued fever, considerable difference of opinion has prevailed. Dr. Heberden cautiously observes: "I am not so sure of its being useful, as I am of its being innocent." In order to avoid offending the stomach, it is frequently advisable to begin with the infusion, for which, afterwards, first the decoction, then the sulphate of quina, may be substituted. In the stage of convalescence, the use of cinchona or sulphate of quina may often be advantageously preceded by infusion of calumba; without this precaution, irritation of the stomach or febrile symptoms are readily set up.

8. *In inflammatory diseases.*– As a general rule, stimulants and tonics, as cinchona, are improper in inflammatory diseases. Yet to this statement, which applies principally to the first stage, to acute and active cases, and to the disease when it occurs in strong and vigorous habits, many exceptions exist. Thus, when it takes place in old and debilitated constitutions; when it is of a mild or atonic character, and

has existed for some time without giving rise to any obvious organic changes; when it assumes an intermittent or even remittent form; or when it is of a certain quality, which experience has shown to be less benefited by ordinary antiphlogistic measures, cinchona is sometimes admissible and advantageous after evacuations have been made proportioned to the activity of the disease and the vigour of the system. *In scrofulous inflammation* (as of the eye) its value is fully appreciated. *In rheumatism,* in which disease Morton, Fothergill, Saunders, and Haygarth have so strongly recommended it, its use is now obsolete, except under circumstances similar to those which regulate its employment in ordinary inflammation. The same remarks apply to its employment in *erpsiyelatous inflammation,* in which it was at one time much esteemed.

4. *In maladies characterized by atony and debility.–* Cinchona is useful in a great variety of diseases dependent on, or attended by, a deficiency of tone or strength, as indicated by a soft and lax condition of the solids, weak pulse, incapability of great exertion, impaired appetite, and dyspeptic symptoms. Thus, *in chronic atonic affections of the alimentary canal,* it proves very serviceable, especially in some forms of dyspepsia and anorexia. In these, it should be given half an hour or an hour before meal-times. *In some chronic maladies of the nervous system,* as chorea, when it occurs in delicate girls; also, in the neuralgia of weakly subjects. Disulphate of quina has been used by Dr. Bright' in tetanus. *In mortification,* it is useful in those cases in which tonics and astringents are obviously indicated; but it has no specific power of checking the disease, as was formerly supposed. *In passive hemorrhages,* from relaxation of vessels, as in some cases of profuse menstruation, or uterine hemorrhage consequent on miscarriage. *In profuse mucous discharges* with great debility, as in leucorrhoea, excessive bronchial secretion, old diarrhoeas, &c. *In cachectic diseases,* as enlargements and indurations of the absorbent glands, of a scrofulous nature, strumous ophthalmia, obstinate ulcers, &c. Also in venereal diseases, when the secondary symptoms occur in shattered and broken-down constitutions, and after the full use of mercury. Likewise in some of the chronic skin diseases, which are seen in cachectic habits.

5. *In the convalescence* of either acute or chronic lingering diseases, as fever, inflammation, hemorrhage, profuse suppuration, &c.; also after important surgical operations, when the strength is greatly reduced. In no class of cases is the efficacy of cinchona or its alkaloids more manifest than in these.

6. *As a topical astringent and antispeptic.–* The efficacy of cinchona as an astringent and antispeptic depends on tannic acid. Rut as many vegetable substances exceed cinchona in the quantity of this acid which they contain, so they surpass it in astringency. Hence, the topical uses of bark are comparatively unimportant;

and, for the most part, are nearly obsolete. Powdered cinchona is frequently employed as a tooth-powder. Formerly, it was used as an application to mortified parts, foul ulcers, caries, &c. The decoction, with or without hydrochloric acid, is applied as a gargle in putrid sore throat.

7. *As a chemical antidote.–* The value of cinchona bark, as a chemical antidote, depends on its tannic acid. I have already offered some observations on its employment in poisoning by emetic tartar (see vol. i. p. 670). I believe, in all cases, it might be advantageously replaced by other and more powerful astringents; as nut,galls, or, *on* an emergency, green tea.

Administration.– In the form of *powder,* cinchona is now rarely administered. The bulk of a full dose, its disagreeable taste, its tendency to causa nausea and vomiting, and. the quantity of inert woody fibre which it contains, form great objections to its employment. Yet, of its great efficacy, as a febrifuge or antiperiodic, in intermittents, and of its superiority in these cases to the decoction or infusion, no doubt can exist; but sulphate of quina has almost entirely superseded it. The dose of the powder of cinchona is from a, scruple to a drachm, or even more than this when the stomach can bear it.

The dose of the tincture is one to three fluiddrachm.

Bruce A. Evans, M.D.

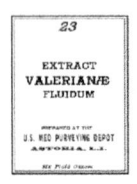

Extract Valerianæ Fluidum - Clear fluid

(Documented use in ancient times)

This is a sedative to the nervous system, most appropriate to the treatment of the milder forms of hysteria and hypochondriasis. The dose is one to three fluidrachms.

Modern Perspective:

This herbal remedy has remained popular through the years and is still easily found in health food and alternative medicine stores.
It is essentially non-toxic, and also probably of little use, although it probably has a very mild sedative effect.

Period Reference:

The Elements of Materia Medica and Therapeutics – Jonathan Pereira, M.D. (Blanchard and Lee, Philadelphia, 1852) on the uses and administration of:

Valerian

Uses.– Valerian may be employed as a nervous excitant, and, where stimulants are admissible, as an antispasmodic. It was formerly in great repute. It has been principally celebrated in *epilepsy*. It came into use in modern times through the recommendation of Fabius Columba, who reported himself cured by it, though it appears he suffered a relapse. Its employment has found numerous advocates and opponents, but at the present time practitioners regard it as a medicine of very little power. In the few cases in which I have employed it, it has failed to give the least relief. In some of the milder and more recent forms of the disease, neither dependent on any lesion within the cranium nor accompanied with plethora' as in hysterical epilepsy, it may occasionally prove serviceable. In *chorea,* and other spasmodic affections, it has been used with variable success. I have found temporary benefit from its use in females affected with *hypochondriasis* and *hysteria.* Of its use as a nervous stimulant in the low forms of *fever,* we have but little experience in this country. In Germany, where it is more esteemed, its employment in these cases is spoken highly of.

Administration. – The dose of the *powder* is from a scruple to a drachm or even two drachm. Though objected to by some on account of the quantity of inert woody fibre which it contains, it is, when well and recently prepared, an efficacious form for administration. The dose of the fluidextract is from 10 to 40 drops.

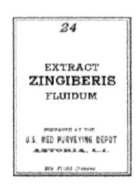

```
    24
  EXTRACT
 ZINGIBERIS
  FLUIDUM

U.S. MED PURVEYING DEPOT
   ASTORIA, L.I.
```

Extract Zingiberis Fluidum (Extract of Ginger Root) - Greenish-blue liquid

This is a mild stimulant in doses of 10 to 20 minims or 20 to 40 drops. It is used mostly for dyspepsia, being helpful to settle the stomach and treat excess gas (flatulence). When added to bitter tonics, it results in increased acceptance and makes the combination easier on the stomach.

Modern Perspective:

This non-toxic substance is essentially medically inactive.

Period Reference:

The Elements of Materia Medica and Therapeutics – Jonathan Pereira, M.D. (Blanchard and Lee, Philadelphia, 1852) on the uses and administration of:
Ginger

Physiological Effects.– Ginger is one of the aromatic stimulants (see vol. i. p. 258) which possess considerable pungency or acridity. Its dust applied to the mucous membrane of the nostrils acts as an irritant, and provokes sneezing. The rhizome chewed is a powerful sialagogue. The powder mixed with hot water, and applied to the skin, causes a sensation of intense heat and tingling, and slight redness. When taken into the stomach, ginger operates as a stimulant; first, to the alimentary canal; secondly, to the body generally; but especially to the organs of respiration. Like some other spices (the peppers, for instance), it acts as an excitant to the genital organs. Furthermore, it has been said to increase the energy of the cerebral functions. It is less acrid than pepper.

Uses.– Its principal consumption is as a *condiment.* Its powers in this way are considerable, while its flavour is by no means disagreeable, and its acridity scarcely sufficient to enable it, when taken with food, to irritate or inflame.

As a *stomachie* and *internal stimulant,* it serves several important purposes. In enfeebled and relaxed habits, especially of old and gouty individuals, it promotes digestion, and relieves flatulency and spasm of the stomach and bowels. It checks or prevents nausea and griping, which are apt to be produced by some drastic purgatives. It covers the nauseous flavour of many medicines, and communicates cordial and carminative qualities to tonic and other agents. As a *sialagogue,* it is sometimes chewed to relieve toothache, relaxed uvula, and paralytic affections of the tongue. As a *counter-irritant,* I have frequently known a *ginger plaster* (prepared .by mixing together powdered ginger and warm water, and spreading the paste on paper or cloth) relieve violent headache when applied to the forehead.

Administration.– *Powdered ginger* may be administered, in doses of from ten grains to a scruple or more, in the form of a pill. Made into a paste with hot water, it may be applied as a *plaster,* as already mentioned.

Preserved ginger (conditum zinpiberis), though commonly used as a sweetmeat, may be taken with advantage as a medicine to stimulate the stomach. Ginger *lozenges, ginger pearls* (commonly termed *ginger seeds),* and *ginger pipe* are useful articles of confectionery, which are frequently of benefit in dyspepsia accompanied with flatulence.

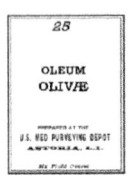

Oleum Olivæ (olive oil) -
Pale yellow or greenish yellow thick liquid

Externally, olive oil is used to relax skin, protect lesions from the air, and as a compounding vehicle for active substances in liniments, ointments, cerates, and plasters. May be used internally as a mild laxative in irritative disorders when the patient objects to the use of stronger agents.

Modern Perspective:

This non-toxic substance is essentially medically inactive.

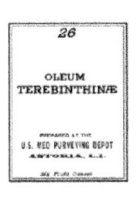

Oleum Terebinthinæ (oil of turpentine) -
Colorless liquid

   This is used externally to bring color and warmth to the skin in fever with clammy skin, applied with soaked flannel strips (stupes). Used internally, it causes prompt expulsion of worms.

Modern Perspective:

   This irritative substance was used to provoke an inflammatory reaction on the skin.

   The presumed benefits of that reaction, in reducing pathologic inflammation in a contiguous area ("counter-irritation") or a distant site ("revulsion"), postulated from the theory that the patient's "system" could only sustain a fixed amount of inflammation and vascular excitement, are illusory.

   The internal use to kill and/or expel parasitic worms does appear to have that effect: such use persists as a folk remedy as well as in "natural" vetinary use, especially for swine. Its use in general however has been superceded by more modern remedies due to the toxicity when used internally, which ranges from pain and burning to to local irritation to central nervous system depression causing initial excitement, then incoordination, delirium, coma, respiratory depression and death with a mean lethal dose of 4-6 ounces.

Period Reference:

Bruce A. Evans, M.D.

The Elements of Materia Medica and Therapeutics – Jonathan Pereira, M.D. (Blanchard and Lee, Philadelphia, 1852) on the uses and administration of:

Oil of Turpentine

Uses.– The following are the principal uses of the oil of turpentine: –

1. As *an anthelmintic.*– *It* is the most effectual remedy for *tape-worm* we possess. It both causes the death of, and, expels the parasite from the body. To adults it should be given in doses of an ounce at least. I have frequently administered an ounce and a half, and sometimes two ounces. Occasionally, as in Dr. Copland's case, it fails to purge, but becoming absorbed, operates most severely on the system, causing disorder of the cerebral functions. It is said to be more apt to act thus in persons of a full and plethoric habit. To prevent these ill consequences, an oleaginous purgative should be either conjoined with it, or given at an interval of four or five hours after it. An excellent and safe method of employing it is to combine it with a castor-oil emulsion. *Chabert's empyreumatic oil* (described at vol. i. p. 268) used by Bremser against tape-worm, consists principally of oil of tur- pentine. A very effectual remedy for the *small thread-worm (Ascaris vermicularis)* is the turpentine enema.

2. *In blennorrhea.*– Oil of turpentine sometimes checks or stops profuse chronic discharges from the mucous membranes. It appears to effect this by a topical influence over the capillary and secerning vessels, in its passage through them out of the system. In many cases, it would appear to confine its operation to the production of an increase of tonicity in the vessels which pour out mucus; but in other instances, especially in blennorrhoea of the urinary apparatus, it seems to set up a new kind of irritation in the affected membrane, which supersedes the previously existing disease. Hence its use is not admissible in acute or recent affections of these tissues. In gonorrhea and gleet I have frequently employed it as a substitute for balsam of copaiba with success. In leucorrhoea it has occasionally proved serviceable. In catarrhus vesicle or cystirrhoea, it now and then acts

beneficially; but it requires to be used in small doses and with great caution. In chronic pulmonary catarrh, either mucous or pituitous, it is said to have been employed with advantage- In chronic diarrhoea and dysentery it has proved advantageous: in these cases it has a direct local action on the affected part, besides exerting its influence over *this* in common with other mucous membranes after its absorption.

3. *In hemorrhages.–* In sanguineous exhalations, called hemorrhages, from the mucous surfaces, oil of turpentine may, under some circumstances, act efficaciously. On the same principle that it checks excessive secretion of mucus in catarrhal conditions of these tissues, so we can readily conceive it may stop the exhalation of blood. But it is only admissible in cases of a passive or atonic character, in the absence of plethora and a phlogistic diathesis. In purpura haemorrhagica it has been recommended as a purgative, by Dr. Whitlock Nichol, Dr. Magee, and others. I have seen it act injuriously in this disease, while blood-letting has seemed to relieve.

4. *In puerperal fever.–* The use of the oil of turpentine as a specific in this disease was introduced by Dr. Brenan, of Dublin, and strong testimonies were subsequently borne to its effcacy by several highly respectable practitioners. Dr. Brenan gave one or two tablespoonfuls of the oil, every three or four hours, in cold water, sweetened; and applied flannel soaked in the oil to the abdomen. But the apparent improbability of a stimulant like turpentine curing an inflammatory disease, has prevented many practitioners placing any faith in it, or even giving it a trial. In other instances, the unconquerable aversion which patients have manifested to it has precluded its repetition. Lastly, it has failed, in the hands of some of our most accurate observers, to produce the good effects which Dr. Brenan and others have ascribed to it, and in some instances has appeared to aggravate the malady. These reasons have been conclusive against its employment, at least in the way advised by Dr. Brenan. But there are two valuable uses which may be made of turpentine, in puerperal fever: it may be given in the form of clyster, to relieve a tympanitic condition of the intestines, and for this purpose no remedy perhaps is superior to it; secondly, flannel soaked in the hot oil may be applied

to the abdomen to cause rubefaction, as a substitute for a blister, to the employment of which several objections exist.

5. *In ordinary fever.–* As a powerful stimulant in some forms of low fever, oil of turpentine has been well spoken of by Dr. Holst, Dr. Chapman, Dr. Douglas, and more recently by Dr. Wood. When the skin is dry, the bowels flatulent, and ulceration of the mucous membrane suspected, it often proves most serviceable.

6. *In rheumatism.–* In chronic rheumatism, oil of turpentine has long been celebrated. Its beneficial influence depends on its stimulant and diaphoretic operation, and is more likely to be evinced in old and debilitated persons. I have found medium doses occasionally succeed when small ones have failed. But for the most part I have not met with that success with it in chronic rheumatism, to induce me to place much confidence in it. In the form of liniment it has often proved serviceable.

7. *In sciatica and other neuralgic affections.–* Oil of turpentine was proposed as a remedy for sciatica by Drs. Pitcairn and. G. Cheyne. Its efficacy was subsequently confirmed by Dr. Home. More recently it has been extensively employed, and with great success, in France, in sciatica as well as in various other neuralgias. But it has proved more successful in those which affect the lower extremities. My own experience does not lead me to speak very favourably of it. In a disease the pathology of which is so imperfectly understood as is that of neuralgia, it is vain to attempt any explanation of the *methodus medendi* of an occasional remedy for it. I have known oil of turpentine now and then act most beneficially in sciatica, without giving rise to any remarkable evacuation by the bowels, skin, or kidneys, so that the relief could not be ascribed to a cathartic, a diaphoretic, or a diuretic operation.

8. *In suppression of urine.–* T have seen oil of turpentine succeed in reproducing the urinary secretions when other powerful diuretics had failed.

9. *In infantile diabetes.–* Dr. Dewees has cured three cases of diabetes [?] in infants under fifteen months old. "by keeping the

bowels freely open, and putting a quantity of spirits of turpentine upon the clothes of the children, so as to keep them in a terebinthinate atmosphere."

10. *In nephritic diseases,–* In some diseases of the kidneys, as ulceration, the use of oil of turpentine has been much extolled. It has proved successful in renal hydatids.

11. *In dropsy.–* Oil of turpentine has occasionally proven serviceable in the chronic forms of this disease. Its efficacy depends, in part, on its derivative operation as a stimulating diuretic; and in part, as I conceive, on its powerful influence over the capillary and secerning vessels, by which it exercises a direct power *of* checking effusion. It is inadmissible, or is contraindicated, in dropsies accompanied with arterial excitement, or with irritation of the stomach or the urinary organs. When the effusion depends on obstruction to the return of venous blood, caused by the pressure of enlarged or indurated viscera, tumours, &c., turpentine can be of no avail. But in the atonic forms of dropsy, especially in leucophlegmatic subjects, attended with deficient secretion of the skin and kidneys, this oil is calculated. to be of benefit. Dr. Copland has used it in the stage of turgescence, or invasion of acute hydrocephalus, as a drastic and derivative.

12. *In spasmodic diseases.–* Oil of turpentine has been. employed successfully in the treatment of epilepsy, by Drs. Latham, Young, Ed. Percival, Lithgow, Copland, and Pritchard. No benefit can be expected from this or any other medicine, when the disease depends on organic lesion within the osseous envelope of the nervous centres. But when the disease is what Dr. Marshall Hall terms *centripetal* or *eccentric* (as the convulsion of infants frequently is), that is, takes its origin in parts distant from the cerebro-spinal axis, which becomes affected only through the. incident or excitor nerves, we can easily understand that benefit may be obtained by the use of agents like this, which, while it stimulates the abdominal viscera, operates as a cathartic and anthelmintic, and produces a derivative action on the head. A more extended experience of its use in chorea, hysteria, and tetanus, is requisite to enable us to speak with confidence of its

efficacy in these diseases, though a few successful cases have been published.

18. *In inflammation of the eye.–* Mr. Guthrie has employed oil of turpentine in inflammation of the iris and. choroid coat, on the plan recommended by Mr. Hugh Carmichael. In some cases, especially those of an arthritic nature, it succeeded admirably, in others it was of little or no service. It was given in doses of a drachm three times a day.

14. *In tympanites.–* To relieve flatulent distension of the stomach and bowels, and the colic thereby induced, both in infants and adults, oil of turpentine is a most valuable remedy. It should be given in full doses, so as to act as a purgative; or when, from any circumstance, it cannot be exhibited by the mouth, it may be employed in the form of clyster. Dr. Ramsbotham speaks in the highest terms of the efficacy of the oil of turpentine in the acute tympanites of the puerperal state, and thinks that most of the cases of the so-called puerperal fever, which yielded to this oil, were in fact cases of acute tympanites; and in this opinion he is supported by Dr. Marshall Hall.

15. *In obstinate constipation.–* Dr. Kinglake, in a case of obstinate constipation with a tyrnpanitic condition of the intestines, found oil of turpentine a successful cathartic, after the ordinary means of treating these cases had been assiduously tried in vain. Dr. Paris also speaks highly of it in obstinate constipation depending on affections of the brain.

16. *To assist the passage of biliary calculi.–* A mixture of three parts sulphuric ether and two parts oil of turpentine has been recommended as a solvent for biliary calculi. But there is no foundation for the supposition that the relief which may be obtained by the use of this mixture in icterus, and during the passage of a biliary calculus, depends on the dissolution of the latter.

17. As *an external remedy.–* Oil of turpentine is employed externally, as a *rubefacient,* in numerous diseases, on the principle of counter-irritation, before explained (vol. i p. 170). Thus in the form of liniment, it is used, either hot or cold, in chronic rheummatism,

sprains, sore throat, neuralgic affections of the extremities, &c. In the form of fomentation the hot oil is applied to produce redness of the skin in puerperal peritonitis, as I have already mentioned. As a powerful local *stimulant*, it was recommended by Dr. Kentish as an application to burns and scalds, his object being to restore the part gradually, not suddenly, to its natural state, as in the treatment of a case of frost-bite. The practice is most successful when the local injury is accompanied with great constitutional depression. I can bear testimony to its efficacy in such cases, having employed it in several most severe and dangerous burns with the happiest results. In that form of gangrene which is not preceded by inflammation, and is called *dry* or *chronic*, oil of turpentine may occasionally prove serviceable, especially when the disease affects the toes and feet of old people. There are other topical uses to which it has been applied; but as they are for the most part obsolete, at least in this country, I omit any further mention of them. They are fully noticed in the works of Voigtels and Richter. Oil of turpentine is the principal ingredient in *Whitehead's Essence of Mustard*, which contains also camphor and a portion of the spirits of rosemary. *St. John Long's liniment'* consisted of oil of turpentine and acetic acid, held in suspension by yolk of egg.

Administration.– When given as a diuretic, and to affect the capillary and secerning vessels (in catarrhal affection of the mucous membranes, dropsy, suppression of urine, hemorrhage, &c.) the dose is from six or eight minims to a fluiddrachm; as a general stimulant (in chronic rheumatism, chorea, &c.) or to produce a change in the condition of the intestinal coats (in chronic dysentery), from one to two fluiddrachm; as an anthelmintic (in tape-worm) or as a revulsive (in apoplexy, in epilepsy previous to an expected paroxysm, &c.), from one-half to two fluidounces. It may be taken floating on some hot aromatic water, to which some hot aromatic tincture, as *tinctera capsici,* has been added; or it may be diffused through water by the aid of mucilage or an emulsion; or it may be made into a linctus with honey or some aromatic syrup.

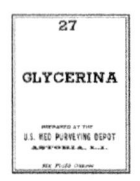

Glycerina (glycerine) -
Straw color syrup

Glycerine may be used on skin lesions as a smoothing emollient. It also has antiseptic properties when applied to skin lesions tending to putrification.

Modern Perspective:

This non-toxic substance is essentially medically inactive.

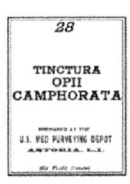

Tinctura Opii Camphorata (camphorated tincture of opium; paregoric) -
Reddish-green liquid

This mixture combines the pain relieving and antidiarrheal effects of **opium** with the anti-spasmodic effects of camphor. As such, at least for limited if not chronic use, it is of benefit in dysentery with diarrhea and accompanying painful abdominal and pelvic spasms. In a dose of 1-2 fluidrachms, it checks diarrhea, relieves nausea, and benefits the abdominal and stomach pains.

Modern Perspective:

The effective component of this medication is the opium, which effectively relieves pain and checks diarrhea (causing constipation with chronic use). Opium in its various forms represented the only effective pain reliever available to the civil war surgeon short of anesthesia.

The camphor was felt to be helpful for so called "spasmodic" disorders, representing abrupt and recurrent events ranging from abdominal cramps to neuralgias to epilepsy. In this preparation it is probably intended to help abdominal cramping, but would not have a significant effect in that regard.

Camphor applied to the skin has a cooling and anti-itching effect.

Period Reference:

Bruce A. Evans, M.D.

The Elements of Materia Medica and Therapeutics – Jonathan Pereira, M.D. (Blanchard and Lee, Philadelphia, 1852) on the uses and administration of:

Camphorated Tincture of Opium

TINCTURA CAMPHORAE COMPOSITA, L.; *Compound Tincture of Opium; Tictura 0pii camphorata,* E. D. [U. S.]; *Elixir Paregoricum; Paregoric Elixir,* offic.– (Camphor 2 and one-half scruples [one drachm, D.]; Opium, powdered [sliced, E.], gr. 72 [one and one-half drachm, D., 4 scuples, E.]; Benzoic Acid gr. 72 [4 scruples, *E.,* one and one-half drachm, D.]; Oil of Anise one fluid ounce; Proof Spirit 2 pints. Macerate for seven days, and filter.) – This is a very valuable preparation, and is extensively employed both by the public and the profession. Its active ingredient is opium. The principal use of it is to allay troublesome cough unconnected with any active inflammatory symptoms. It diminishes the sensibility of the bronchial membrane to the influence of cold air, checks profuse secretion, and allays spasmodic cough. Dose, one to three fluiddrachm. A fluidounce contains nearly two grains of opium. The name given to this preparation by the London College, though less correct than that of the Edinburgh and. Dublin Colleges, is, I conceive, much more convenient, since it enables us to prescribe opium without the knowledge of the patient – no mean advantage in cases where a strong prejudice exists in the mind of the patient or his friends to the use of this important narcotic. Furthermore, it is less likely to give rise to serious and fatal errors in dispensing. In a case mentioned by Dr. M. Good, laudanum was served, by an ignorant dispenser, for *tinct. opii camph.* The error proved fatal to the patient. [For the formula of the *U. S. Pharm.,* see Preparations of Opium.]

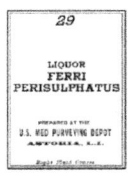

Liquor Ferri Persulphatus (ferric persulphate solute) Bluish-green liquid

The main use of this substance is as a styptic and astringent. This drug causes blood coagulation when applied without causing irritation to the tissues. It may be applied with a hair brush, or with lint for larger areas.

Modern Perspective:

This substance does cause clotting of blood through enhanced coagulation of plasma proteins. It is still used as a styptic preparation, especially in veterinary applications, and is available over the counter in pet shops for treatment of bleeding scratches on cats and dogs and other small animals.
It was not used internally, unlike other iron-based "tonics".

Period Reference:

The Elements of Materia Medica and Therapeutics – Jonathan Pereira, M.D. (Blanchard and Lee, Philadelphia, 1852) on the uses and administration of:
Ferric Perphosphate

The uses and administration of the Persulphate of Iron are similar to those described for the Sulphate:

Uses.– Sulphate of iron is to be preferred to other ferruginous compounds where there is great relaxation of the solid parts, with immoderate discharges. Where the long-continued use of ferruginous compounds is required, it is less adapted for administration than some other preparations of iron, on account of its local action on the alimentary canal.

It is employed in lump, powder, or solution, as a styptic, to check hemorrhage from numerous small vessels. A solution of it is applied to ulcerated surfaces and to mucous membranes to diminish profuse discharges, as in chronic ophthalmia, leucorrhoea, aud gleet. Mr. Vincent used it in prolapsus ani (see *ante,* p. 229). A solution of three drachms of the sulphate in five ounces of water has been used by Velpeau to repress erysipelas.

Internally, it is administered in passive hemorrhages, on account of its supposed astringent influence over the system generally; also in immoderate secretion and exhalation – as in humid asthma, chronic mucous catarrh, old dysenteric affections, colliquative sweating, diabetes, leucorrhoea, gleet, &c. In intermittents, it has been employed as a tonic. It has also been found serviceable against tape-worm. Its other uses are the same as the ferruginous compounds before mentioned.

Administration.– The dose of it is from one to five grains in the form of pill. If given in solution, the water should be recently boiled, to expel the atmospheric air dissolved in it, the oxygen of which converts this salt into a persulphate. A very agreeable method of exhibiting sulphate of iron is in solution in carbonic acid water. Mr. Webb prepared it for me of three strengths; one containing three grains, a second six grains, a third nine grains of the crystallized sulphate to each bottle of carbonic acid water (bottle soda water).

For local purposes, solutions of it are employed of various strengths, according to circumstances. In chronic ophthalmia, we may use one or two grains to an ounce of water; as an injection in gleet, from four to ten grains. It has been used to disinfect night soil; the products are sulphate of ammonia and hydrated sulphuret of iron.

Bruce A. Evans, M.D.

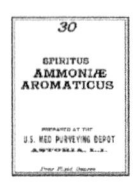

Spiritus Ammoniæ Aromaticus (aromatic spirits of ammonia) - Brownish liquid

This is used as a stimulant, one to two fluidounces diluted in water. It is helpful for languor, hysteria, or nervous disability. It also benefits flatulent colic, which not infrequently accompanies the foregoing symptoms.

Modern Perspective:

The well-known "stimulant" effect of ammonia vapor - "smelling salts" - account for whatever effect this medication brought to bear on the mainly psychosomatic indications for its use - languor, hysteria, or nervous disability. The alcohol content of the tincture probably also played a role.

The toxicity is local esophageal and stomach irritation, and due to the corrosive effect of a concentrated solution.

Period Reference:

The Elements of Materia Medica and Therapeutics – Jonathan Pereira, M.D. (Blanchard and Lee, Philadelphia, 1852) on the uses and administration of:
Aromatic Spirits of Ammonia

1, SPIRITUS AMMONIAE AROMATICUS, L. E. D. [U. S.]; *Spiritus Salis Volatilis Oleosus; Spirit of Sal Volatile.–* The preparation of the London Pharmacopoeia is a solution of the carbonate of ammonia; but those of the Edinburgh and Dublin Pharmacopoeias contain caustic ammonia.

The *London College* gives the following formula: Hydrochlorate of Ammonia 6 ounces; Carbonate of Potash 10 ounces; Cinnamon bruised, Cloves bruised, of each 2 and one half drachms; Lemon Peel 5 ounces; Rectified Spirit, Water, of each 4 pints. Mix them, and let six pints distil.

In this process double decomposition takes place, as already noticed, and the carbonate of ammonia distills over with the spirit and part of the water favoured by the essential oils of the aromatics used. The sp. gr. of this preparation is 0.918.

[The *U. S P.* orders of Muriate of Ammonia five ounces; Carbonate of Potassa eight ounces; Cinnamon bruised, Cloves bruised, each two drachms; Lemon Peel four ounces; Alcohol, Water, each five pints. Mix them, and distil seven pints and a half.]

Prepared according to the London Pharmacopceia, its sp. gr. is 0.018; according to the Dublin Pharmacopoeia, 0.852. It is frequently employed in languor, fainting, hysteria, flatulent colic, and nervous debility, in doses of from one-half to two fluid ounces properly diluted with water.

Uses.– Ammonia is adapted for speedily rousing the action of the vascular and respiratory systems, and for the prompt alleviation of spasm. It is more especially fitted for fulfilling these indications when our object is at the same time to promote the action of the skin. It is calculated for states of debility with torpor or inactivity. It is also used. as an antacid and. local irritant.

1. *In dyspeptic complaints, accompanied with preternatural acidity of stomach and flatulence,* but without inflammation, a properly diluted solution of ammonia may be employed with a twofold object – that of neutralizing the free acid, and, of stimulating the stomach. It must be remembered that the healthy secretions of the stomach are of

an acid nature, and. that the continued use of ammonia, or any other alkali, must ultimately be attended with injurious results, more especially to the digestive functions. While, therefore, the occasional employment of alkalies maybe serviceable, their constant or long-continued use must ultimately prove deleterious.

Ammonia may, under some circumstances, be employed to neutralize acids intro-duced into the stomach from without, as in poisoning by the mineral acids; though chalk and magnesia would be more appropriate, being less irritant. It is a valuable antidote in poisoning by hydrocyanic acid. Its beneficial operation has been ascribed to the union of the alkali with the acid, whereby hydrocyanate of ammonia is formed; but since it has been found. that this salt is highly poisonous, it is evident that this statement cannot be correct. Some have ascribed the activity of the hydrocyanate to its decomposition by the free acids of the stomach, and the consequent evolution of free hydrocyanic acid; but this explanation is not satisfactory. I believe the effeciency of ammonia as an antidote to poisoning by hydrocyanic acid arises from its exerting an influence of an opposite nature to that of the poison. In poisoning by the oil of bitter almonds, or other agents supposed to contain this acid, ammonia is equally serviceable. The antidote should be given by the stomach, if the patient can swallow, and the vapour should be cautiously inhaled.

2. *Ammonia is given internally as a stimulant and sudorific* with manifest advantage in several cases, of which the following are illustrations: –

a. In continued fevers which have existed for some time, and where all violent action has subsided, and the brain does not appear much disordered, it is occasion-ally of great service. Its diaphoretic action should be promoted by diluents and warm clothing. It has an advantage over opium – that, if it do no good, it is less likely to do harm.

b. In intermittent fevers it; is sometimes of advantage, given, during the cold stage, to hasten its subsidence.

c. In the exanthemata, when the eruption has receded from the skin, and the extremities are cold, it is sometimes of great benefit, on account of its stimulant and diaphoretic properties. But in some of these cases the recession arises from, or is connected with, an inflammatory condition of the bronchial membrane, for which the usual treatment is to be adopted.

d. In some inflammatory diseases (especially pneumonia and rheumatism), where the violence of the vascular action has been reduced by proper evacuations, and where the habit of the patient is unfavourable to the loss of blood, ammonia has been serviceable. In combination with decoction of senega, I have found' it valuable in old pulmonary affections. (See *Senega.*)

3. *In certain affections of the nervous system,* ammonia is frequently employed with the greatest benefit. Thus it has been used to relieve the cerebral disorder of intoxication. In poisoning by those cerebro-spinants commonly termed sedatives– such as foxglove, tobacco, and hydrocyanic acid – ammonia is a most valuable agent. This remedy has been supposed to possess a specific influence in relieving those disorders of the nervous system accompanied with spasmodic or convulsive symptoms: and hence it is classed among the remedies denominated *antispasmodic.* Velsen, of Cleves, has used it with advantage in delirium tremens. It was a remedy frequently tried in the malignant or Indian cholera, and occasionally procured relief, but it was not much relied on.

Effects.– The effects of the carbonates of ammonia are similar to, but milder than, those of pure or caustic ammonia (see *ante,* p. 429); and they are milder in proportion as the quantity of carbonic acid they contain is greater. The neutral or monocarbonate, therefore, is more powerful than the sesquicarbonate, and this than the bicarbonate.

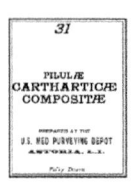

Pillulæ Catharticæ Compositæ (compound cathartic pills)
White solid

This medication is a compound of extract of colocynth and extract of jalap and calomel and gamhose, resulting in cumulative action at smaller doses than the effective laxative dose of each component. The relatively mild but sure action and the small bulk result from this combination. This is the first choice for simple constipation.

Modern Perspective:

This medication is a compound of extract of colocynth and extract of jalap and calomel and gamhose.

Each of these components, with the exception of the calomel, is an energetic purgative. For the production of evacuation in constipation, it certainly would have a dramatic effect. The colocynth in particular can cause dangerous bowel inflammation, leading a times to shock and death. This preparation, with smaller doses than those used of the individual components, would be somewhat less dangerous. The calomel, a weak purgative at best, can lead to dangerous mercury toxicity, since it is a salt form that is readily absorbed.

To the extent that purgation was being used as a means of "counter-irritation" or "revulsion" to treat inflammatory disease elsewhere, or to clean the bowels of postulated retained and toxic substances in dysentery, its use is counterproductive and ineffective.

Period Reference:

The Elements of Materia Medica and Therapeutics – Jonathan Pereira, M.D. (Blanchard and Lee, Philadelphia, 1852) on the uses and administration of:
PILULAE CATHARTICAE COMPOSITAE, Ph. of the United States

Compound Cathartic Pills.– (Compound Extract of Colocynth one-half ounce; Extract of Jalap, in powder, Calomel, of each 3 drachms; Gamboge, in powder, two scruples. M. Divide into 180 pills.) – This pill is intended to combine smallness of bulk with efficiency and comparative mildness of purgative action, and a peculiar tendency to the biliary organs. Each pill contains one grain of calomel. Three pills are a full dose.

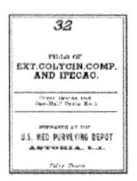

Pills of Ext. Colycyn. Comp. And Ipecac (pills of colocynth compound extract and ipecac)
White solid

The addition of the small dose (½ grain) of ipecac to the energetic but safe purging effect of the 3 grains of colycinth compound extract stimulates the stomach and promotes digestion. It is used in bowel disorders, including obstinate constipation.

Modern Perspective:

This medication is an energetic purgative, due to the effect of the colocynth, which can cause dangerous bowel inflammation, leading a times to shock and death. The addition of the ipecac at this dose would not lead to emesis, but probably would add some gastric irritation to the overall effect.

To the extent that purgation was being used as a means of "counter-irritation" or "revulsion" to treat inflammatory disease elsewhere, or to clean the bowels of postulated retained and toxic substances in dysentery, its use is counterproductive and ineffective.

One and one-half teaspoon of colocynth powder can be fatal.

Period Reference:

The Elements of Materia Medica and Therapeutics – Jonathan Pereira, M.D. (Blanchard and Lee, Philadelphia, 1852) on the uses and administration of:

Colocynth

Uses.– Besides being useful as an ordinary purgative, colocynth is adapted for acting as a stimulus to the abdominal and pelvic vessels and nerves in cases of torpor or inactivity, and on the principle of counter-irritation already explained for determining from other organs. The objections to its use are acute inflammatory affections of the alimentary canal, diseases of the large intestine, &c. The following are the principal cases in which it is employed.: –

1. *In habitual constipation.*– As an ordinary purgative for keeping the bowels regular, the compound extract of colocynth is in common use both among the public and medical men. It operates mildly, certainly, and effectually. I am acquainted with individuals who have taken this substance for years without suffering any inconvenience therefrom. The simple extract is sometimes employed as a substitute but is less advantageous.

2. *In alvine obstruction.*– In some cases of obstinate constipation, with sickness, and other symptoms of an extremely irritable stomach, the compound extract of colocynth occasionally proves invaluable. Occupying but a small bulk, it is retained on the stomach, and succeeds in producing alvine evaluations, where the ordinary liquid purgatives fail, in consequence of being vomited up. Doubtful cases of intussusception and hernia, even with stercoraceous vomiting, I have seen completely relieved by it. More than once have I known an operation averted by its use, in those who, in addition to the above symptoms, had old hernia, which led the surgeon to suspect strangulation. A slight degree of abdominal tenderness is not to be considered as absolutely prohibiting its use. Occasionally, the extract, is rubbed down with soap and water, and administered as an enema (see *Enema Colocynthydis).*

3. *In diseases of the brain.*– In apoplexy, or a tendency thereto, in paralysis, insanity, violent headache, &c., colocynth is sometimes employed with good. effect, on the principle of revulsion or counter-irritation.

4. *In dropsy.–* In dropsical affections, colocynth has been used as a hy*dragogue. B*ut in this country it is less frequently employed for this than for other purposes; various other hydragogues (especially elaterium and jalap) being usually preferred. It is sometimes employed as a *diuretic,* being given in the form of decoction. Hufeland regarded it as a most effectual diuretic in persons of a cold and sluggish habit of body.

5. *In amenorrhoea, and chlorosis.–* In some cases of obstructed menstruation, beneit is obtained by the use of drastic purgatives, like colocynth, which act on the rectum, and, by contiguous sympathy, affect the uterus.

Administration.– The *powder* which is rarely used, may be administered in doses of from two to eight or ten grains, intimately mixed with some mild powder (gum, or starch). The *decoction* (prepared by boiling 2 drachms of colocynth in one pint of water for six minutes, and, according to Hufeland, adding to the strained liquor 2 drachms of the spirit of sulphuric ether, and one fluid ounce of syrup of orange-peel) is given in doses of one-half fluid ounce three times a day. The *tincture* (prepared according to the Prussian pharmacopceia, by digesting one ounce of colocynth pulp and one ounce of star anise, in one quart of rectified spirit) is given in doses of twenty drops. Colocynth has been employed, intraleptically by Dr. Chrestien. The tincture of colocynth, or an ointment consisting of twenty grains of the powder mixed with hogslard, has been used by way of friction on the abdomen and inner side of the thighs, in disorders of the intellectual functions.

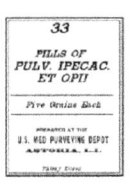

Pills of Pulvis Ipecac et Opii (5 grain pills of powder of ipecac and opium, ½ grain each with 4 grains potassa sulphate; Dover's Powder)
White pills

In doses of 5 - 15 grains every 4 to 8 hours, these pills are used for sthenic diseases such as acute rheumatism and pneumonia. The opium provides pain relief, and the addition of the ipecac results in greatly enhanced sweating, benefiting both the hot, dry skin and creating a revulsive impression to the skin, thereby benefiting the inflammation. Due to the constipating effect, the use of this medicine should be preceded by a mild purge. This medicine may be usefully combined with **calomel** in bowel diseases associated with inflammation.

Modern Perspective:

The vomiting induced by ipecac is probably due both the irritation of the stomach and a central nervous system effect. Poisoning is rare; when it occurs it is due to persistent violent vomiting and bloody diarrhea leading to shock and death.

In a non-addict, 10 grains (600mg.) of opium may be fatal, due to depression of the central nervous system with coma, pinpoint pupils, and respiratory depression. It may also cause fluid to build up in the lungs.

This combination did relieve pain - opium and its derivatives were the only effective pain medications known. The effect of increasing perspiration fit in with theories of disease and symptom treatment, but had no benefical effect on the dieases being treated.

Period Reference:

The Elements of Materia Medica and Therapeutics – Jonathan Pereira, M.D. (Blanchard and Lee, Philadelphia, 1852) on the uses and administration of:

PULVIS IPECACUANHAE COMPOSITUS, L E D.;
Compound powder of Ipeca cuanha; Dover's Powder; Pulvis Doveri, offic. *(Pulvis Ipecacuanha* et *Opii, U.* S.) – (Ipecacuanha, powdered, Hard Opium, powdered, of each one drachm; Sulphate of Potash, powdered, one ounce. Mix them. The proportions used by all the British colleges are the same.) – This preparation is an imitation (though not a very exactone) of a formula given by Dover, whence it is commonly known in the shops as *Dover's Powder.*

The compound powder of ipecacuanha is one of our most certain, powerful, and valuable sudorifics. The sulphate of potash is intended to serve the double purpose of promoting the sudorific operation of the other ingredients, and of minutely dividing, by the hardness of its particles, the opium and ipecacuanha. The nitrate of potash also employed by Dr. Dover probably contributed still further to the sudorific effect of the powder. The opium and ipecaeuanha, combined, enjoy great sudorific properties not possessed by either of these substances individually. I am inclined, however, to ascribe the greater part of the activity of the compound to the opium, which, it is well known, strongly determines to the cutaneous surface (see Opium), and often produces pricking or itching of the skin; and, when assisted by the copious use of warm aqueous diluents, operates as a sudorific. This effect, however, is greatly promoted by the ipecacuanha, which has a relaxing influence over the cutaneous vessels. The use of the posset, enjoined by Dr. Dover, is an important part of the sudorific plan. The contra-indications for the use of compound powder of ipecacuanha are an irritable condition of the stomach (when this preparation is apt to occasion sickness) and cerebral disorder. Thus, in fever, a dry furred tongue, and a dry skin, with much disorder of the cerebro-spinal functions, it, like other opiates, is calculated to prove injurious. In such cases, the antimonial sudorifics may be resorted to. But when the tongue is moist, the skin, if not damp, at least soft – and the functions of the brain not much involved, it will probably operate beneficially. In slight colds, catarrhs, and rheumatic pains, it often proves most effectual. In various inflammatory affections, when the febrile excitement does not run too high, and when the brain is undisturbed, it may be used with good effect. In acute rheumatism it is occasionally highly serviceable; in diarrhoea and. dysentery also. In hemorrhages from internal organs, as the uterus, it is useful on the principle of revulsion or counter-irritation, by its power of deter- mining to the skin. The dose of this preparation is usually from grs. 5 to grs. 10, given in currant jelly or gruel, or made into a pill (see *Pilulm Ipecaceanhe et Opii),* or administered in a common saline draught. Where the stomach is irritable, I have frequently seen five grains cause sickness. On the other hand, in some cases where a powerful sudorific is required, and the head quite free, grs. 15 or even a drachm, of this powder are not unfrequently given.

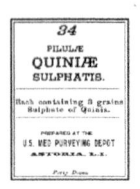

```
       34
     PILULÆ
    QUINIÆ
    SULPHATIS.
  Each containing 3 grains
     Sulphate of Quinia.
    PREPARED AT THE
  U.S. MED PURVEYING DEPOT
     ASTORIA, L.I.
        Forty Doses
```

Pilulæ Quinine Sulphatus (Quinine sulphate pills, 3 grains each)
Yellow pills

(This was purified and identified as the anti-intermittent principle of cinchona bark in 1820)

This medication is an absolute specific for intermittent fever, when this is carefully defined. It is given during the interval between paroxysms of fever in doses sufficient to prevent subsequent episodes (up to 20 grains at a dose). Its use in other forms of fever is less sure. Large doses cause roaring or ringing in the ears; larger doses cause dizziness and occasionally delirium.

Modern Perspective:

The active ingredient of cinchonas - quinine - is an effective treatment of malaria. In the early to mid-19th century, it was recognized that a disease characterized by severe bouts of fever and delirium ending in drenching sweats, occurring at very regular and therefore predictable intervals with no fever in-between could be effectively treated with preparations of cinchona bark, and even more effectively by the purified ingredient quinine.

The bark and its derivatives were therefore felt to be an effective treatment for febrile disease in general, although it was discovered soon enough that patients with other fever patterns such as continued fever (steady or mildly fluctuating), hectic (a fever swinging irregularly and wildly to high values), or remittent (periodic but not returning to normal between not so predictable and regular attacks) did not respond. We know now that quinine directly attacks the blood cell parasite that causes malaria - "intermittent fever" - but does not have a generalized effect on the other diseases causing the noted fever patterns, and does not have a fever-lowering effect as do aspirin, ibuprofen, and similarly more modern anti-inflammatory drugs.

Period Reference:

The Elements of Materia Medica and Therapeutics – Jonathan Pereira, M.D. (Blanchard and Lee, Philadelphia, 1852) on the uses and administration of:

See entry for Tinctura Cinchonas Fluidum

Comparison of the Effects of the Cinchona Bark with their Alkaloids.– It has been asserted that the cinchona alkaloids (i.e., quinine) possess all the medicinal properties of the barks and may be substituted for them on every occasion; but I cannot subscribe *to* either of these statements; for, in the first place, the alkaloids are deficient in the aromatic quality possessed by the barks, and which assists them to sit easily on the stomach; and it is to this circumstance that I am disposed to refer a fact which I have often observed, that sulphate of quina will sometimes irritate the stomach, occasion nausea and pain, and give rise to febrile symptoms, while the infusion of bark is retained without the least uneasiness. Moreover, we must not overlook the tannic acid, which confers on bark an astringent property. So, that while we admit that the essential tonic operation of the barks depends on the alkaloids which they contain, yet the latter are not always equally efficacious. In some cases however, they are of great advantage, since they enable us to obtain, in a small volume, the tonic operation of a large quantity of bark.

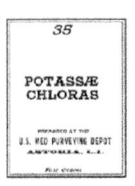

Potassæ Chloras (potassium chlorate) –
White salt

This salt brings down fever while mildly increasing urination, benefiting sthenic fevers. As such it may be used in intermittent or continued fever, especially in later stage of dry skin and scanty urine to increase sweating and urination. It seems to have an beneficial effect on the blood of uncertain cause (alterative effect) in certain low febrile diseases associated with inflammation but depraved or putrid condition of the blood, including typhoid, putrid ulceration and gangrene, scurvy, late stages of smallpox, and malignant erysipelas. When ulcers or gangrene are present, it can be used both internally and as a wash. The dose is 10 to 30 grains in 2 to 3 fluidounces of water.

Modern Perspective:

This is one of several salts used for the general effect of promoting sweating and good urine output. This was felt to benefit many febrile diseases since it was noticed that hot, dry skin and a lack of urine output charactered the severe stages of the disease, and that recovery was often heralded by a drenching sweat as the fever "broke" and recovery was followed by a restoration of urine output.

This salt in particular, was also felt to have some peculiar power to deliver oxygen to the tissues.

None of these effects benefit a disease state, other than those due to the provision of water to an often-dehydrated patient. The combination of fever and dehydration are usually responsible for the dry skin and lack of urine output, and these salts contain nothing having any specific effect.

Potassium, if taken in large doses and not vomited due to gastric irritation, may cause sudden and potentially fatal heart rhythm abnormalities. This is unlikely to happen if the person's kidneys are healthy as potassium is rapidly excreted in that circumstance.

Period Reference:

The Elements of Materia Medica and Therapeutics – Jonathan Pereira, M.D. (Blanchard and Lee, Philadelphia, 1852) on the uses and administration of:

Potassium Chlorate

Uses – Chlorate of potash was originally employed as a medicine for supplying oxygen to the system where a deficiency of that principle was supposed to exist. With that view it was successfully administered by Dr. Garnett in a case of chronic scorbutus. Dr. Ferriar also tried it in scurvy with success. It was subsequently applied in the venereal disease and liver complaints as a substitute for mercurials, whose beneficial effects were thought to depend on the oxygen which they communicated to the system. It has also been tried in cases of general debility, on account of its supposed tonic effects, but failed in the hands of Dr. Ferriar. In a case of dropsy under the care of the latter gentleman, it operated successfully as a diuretic. More recently, it has been used by Dr. Stevens and others as a remedy for fever, cholera, and other malignant diseases, which, he supposes, depend on a deficiency of saline matters in the blood; but, as it is usually employed in conjunction with common salt and carbonate of soda (see *ante,* p. 219), it is impossible to determine what share the chlorate had in producing the beneficial effects said to have been obtained by what is called the *saline* treatment of these diseases. Kohler tried it in phthisis, without experiencing benefit from it.

It appears, then, that most of the uses of this salt have been founded on certain views of chemical pathology, some of which are now considered untenable. It is very desirable, therefore, that some person, unbiassed by theoretical opinions, would carefully investigate its effects and uses, which I am inclined to think have been much overrated. In a therapeutical point of view it may be regarded as analogous to nitrate of potash; though by some it is considered to hold an intermediate position between nitre and sal ammoniac.

It is sometimes employed in scarlatina and cynanche maligna. Frequently it is administered in conjunction with hydrochloric acid as a source of chlorine (see *Mistura et Gargarisma Chlorinii* p. 383)

Cotton wool impregnated with a concentrated solution has been employed as a moxa

Administration - The usual dose of it is from ten or fifteen grains to half a drachm. Dr. Wittmann, in one case, gave 160 grains daily, with a little hydrochloric arid immediately after it, to decompose it. The effects were hot skin; headache; quick, full, and. hard pulse; white tongue; and augmentation of urine.

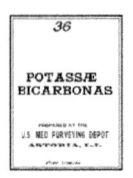

Potassæ Bicarbonas (potassium bicarbonate) -
Colorless, transparent crystals

Used as an antacid in dyspepsia, a diuretic in dropsy, and an antilithic in gravel (kidney and bladder stones) in a dose of 20 grains to a drachm in water solution. It is also used in a weak solution of 2 scruples in water every two hours for acute rheumatism.

Modern Perspective:

The bicarbonate would be of benefit to abdominal distress due to excess stomach acid. In a person with healthy kidneys, the potassium would be non-toxic due to rapid excretion in the urine; if allowed to accumulate dangerous heart rhythm abnormalities may occur.

Period Reference:

The Elements of Materia Medica and Therapeutics – Jonathan Pereira, M.D. (Blanchard and Lee, Philadelphia, 1852) on the uses and administration of: Potassium Bicarbonate

Physiological Effects.– The effects of this salt are similar to those of the carbonate of potash, except that its local action is much less energetic, in consequence of the additional equivalent of carbonic acid. Hence it is an exceedingly eligible preparation in lithiasis (see *ante,* p. 286) and other cases where we want its constitutional, and not its local, action.

Uses.– It may be employed for the same purposes as caustic potash, except that of acting as an escharotic. Thus it is used as an antacid, to modify the quality of urine, in plastic inflammation, in glandular diseases, affections of the urinary organs, &c. It is the active ingredient of a popular lithonlytic called *constitution water.* But its most frequent use is that for ma.king effervescing draughts, with either citric or tartaric acid. The proportions are as follows: –

20 grs. of crystallized Bicarbonate of Potash are saturated by about:

14 grs of commercial crystals of Citric Acid,

15 grs. of crystallized Tartaric Acid,

3 and one-half drachms of Lemon Juice.

Where there is great irritability of stomach, I believe the effervescing draught, made with bicarbonate of potash and citric acid, to be more efficacious than that made with carbonate of soda and tartaric acid. The citrate of potash which is formed promotes slightly the secretions of the alimentary canal, the cutaneous transpiration, and the renal secretion; and, like other vegetable salts of potash, renders the urine alkaline.

Administration.– This salt may be given in doses of from gr. 10 to gr. 15, or to the extent of half a drachm, or even a drachm.

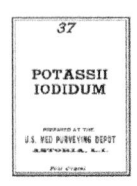

Potassii Iodidum (iodide of potassium) -
Opaque white or transparent crystal

This is used in a dose of 3 grains to one-half ounce, mainly as an expectorant and to increase bronchial secretions in respiratory disease. It has also been found to resolve goiterous tumors, and may benefit scrofula, leucorrhea, and rheumatism of the joints when applied locally in solution.

Modern Perspective:

Iodide solutions have the effect of resolving goiters (swollen thyroid glands) where the reason for the swelling of the gland is a lack of iodine in the diet. Extrapolating from this observed effect, 19th century medicine postulated a "resolvent" effect of reducing the size of abnormal growths of various sorts. Lacking the specific physiologic link to thyroid gland function, this effect is, of course, lacking.

Iodide salts may have a mild expectorant effect on the lungs. The salts are basically non-toxic.

Period Reference:

The Elements of Materia Medica and Therapeutics – Jonathan Pereira, M.D. (Blanchard and Lee, Philadelphia, 1852) on the uses and administration of:
Potassium Iodide

Uses.– Having so fully detailed (see *ante*, p. 899 *et seq.*) the uses of iodine, it is unnecessary to notice at any length those of iodide of potassium, since they are for the most part identical. Thus it has been employed in bronchocele, scrofula, in chronic diseases accompanied with induration and enlargement of various organs, in leucorrhoea, secondary syphilis, periostitis, articular rheumatism, dropsies, &c. As a remedy for the hard periosteal node brought on by syphilis, it was first employed by Dr. Williams, who obtained with it uniform success. At the end of from five to ten days its mitigating effects are felt; the pains are relieved, the node begins to subside, and in the majority of cases disappears altogether. In these cases Dr. Clendinning has also borne testimony to its efficacy. In the tubercular forms of venereal eruptions Dr. Williams found it beneficial. In Dr. Wallace's lectures are some valuable observations on the use of iodide of potassium in venereal diseases. In chronic rheumatism accompanied with alteration in the condition of the textures of the joint, it is, in some cases, remarkably successful. As an ingredient for baths, Lugol found the iodide would not answer alone, but that it was useful as a solvent means for iodine.

Administration.– Iodide of potassium may be employed alone or in conjunction with iodine, forming what is called ioduretted iodide of potassium. *Internally* it has been given alone in doses varying from three grains to half an ounce (see below). To be beneficial, some think it should be given in small, others in large doses. Not having had any experience of the effects of the enormous doses before referred to, I can offer no opinion thereon. The usual dose which I am in the habit of giving to adults is five grains. It may be administered dissolved in simple or medicated water, or in some bitter infusion. It is frequently administered in combination with iodine.

Antidotes.– No chemical antidote is known. In a case of poisoning, therefore, the first object will be to evacuate the contents of the stomach, exhibit demulcent and emollient drinks, combat the inflammation by the usual antiphlogistic measures, and appease the pain by opiates.

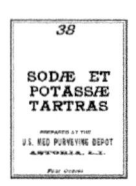

Sodæ et Potassæ Tartras (tartrate of potassium and soda; Rochelle Salt)
Colorless, transparent, large crystal, slightly efflorescent

When used as a mild purgative in a dose of ½ to 1 ounce diluted in water, it also has a cooling effect. It is therefore useful to make an impression on sthenic febrile disorders without harsh effects on the bowels.

Modern Perspective:

This substance is non-toxic in a patient with healthy kidneys so that the potassium is promptly excreted.
This salt in water solution probably had no more effect than to cause a mild looseness of the bowels and a "cooling" taste. As a treatment of inflammatory disease, it it harmless but ineffective.

Period Reference:

The Elements of Materia Medica and Therapeutics – Jonathan Pereira, M.D. (Blanchard and Lee, Philadelphia, 1852) on the uses and administration of:
Tartrate of Potassium and Sodae

Physiological Effects.– It is a mild, laxative, cooling salt, very analogous in its effects to the tartrate of potash. Sundelin says it is uncertain as a purgative – sometimes failing, at others acting very slowly, but strongly, and with violent abdominal pain. He thinks it may be completely replaced in practice by a mixture of magnesia and sulphate of magnesia. When given in the form of dilute solution, and so as not to excite purging, it becomes absorbed, and renders the urine alkaline (see *ante,* p. 218, for a notice of Laveran and Millon's experiments). Hence its use should. be carefully avoided in persons suffering with phosphatic deposits in the urine.

Uses.– It is commonly employed as a mild aperient for females and other delicate persons. It may be used with advantage by those who are subject to excessive secretion of lithic acid or the lithates.

Administration.– It is given in doses of from two to six drachms or an ounce. It should be exhibited largely diluted with water. A very convenient mode of exhibition is in combination with bicarbonate of soda and tartaric acid in an effervescing condition (vide *Seidlitz Powders,* p. 528).

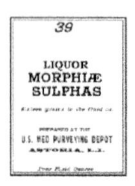

Liquor Morphiæ Sulphas (morphine sulphate solution, 16 gr. to fluidounce)
Whitish liquid

This is a fluid preparation of the main active ingredient in opium, having the same anodyne, perspiration inducing, and sleep producing qualities, but having less stimulating effect, and less after effects of nausea and headache. This form is also often better tolerated by the stomach, and may be used when opium preparations are not retained in the stomach. The usual dose is 1-2 fluidrachms. This form may also be injected under the skin with a syringe and needle, when the medication may not be taken by mouth. This also has the advantage of a faster onset of action.

Modern Perspective:

Morphine sulphate effectively relieves pain and checks diarrhea (causing constipation with chronic use). Opium in its various forms represented the only effective pain reliever available to the civil war surgeon short of anesthesia. Morphine is still the gold standard for pain relief.

The liquid morphine preparation was also beginning to be used subcutaneously by syringe, giving an advantage of a faster onset of action and a smaller dose than medication by mouth.

The civil war surgeon was hampered by the lack of an effective pain reliever for lesser pain. Aspirin was not widely available until the turn of the century for pain and fever relief, although

The Practice of Civil War Medicine and Surgery

folk remedies using bark preparations containing salicylates (related to aspirin) dated back to Native American use.

Period Reference:

The Elements of Materia Medica and Therapeutics – Jonathan Pereira, M.D. (Blanchard and Lee, Philadelphia, 1852) on the uses and administration of:
Morphine Sulphate

Uses.– We employ morphia, or its salts, in preference to opium, when our object is to make applications to the denuded dermis *(endermic medication)*. They are employed in this way for the purpose of alleviating violent neuralgic pains, and to relieve the excessive endermic operation of strychnia. Gastrodynia and obstinate vomiting are sometimes relieved by the endermic application of morphia to the epigastrium; and violent headache by the application of this remedy to the temples. Occasionally, this mode of administration is adopted when we wish to bring the general system under the calming and sedative inhuence of morphia, and where from some cause its exhibition by the mouth is objectionable. Some cases of maniacal delirium may be treated with advantage this way.

The morphia salts are given internally in eases where we wish to obtain the anodyne, soothing, sedative, soporific, and antispasmodic qualities of opium, and where this drug is objectionable on account of its tendency to excite certain injuri-ous effects already referred to. In all cases where both opium and the morphia salts are equally admissible, I prefer the former, its effects being better known and regulated; moreover, opium is to be preferred as a stimulant and sudorific, and for suppressing excessive mucous discharges.

Administration.– The salts are given internally, in a substance or solution, in doses of from one-eighth to one-fourth of a grain, or beyond this. I have given in insanity two grains of muriate of morphia at a dose. For endermic use they are to be finely powdered, and applied to the extent of a grain or a grain and a half at a time.

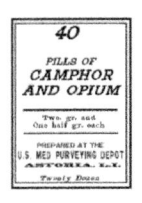

Pills of Camphor and Opium (pills of camphorated opium) - Reddish-green

This medication is similar to paregoric (**Tinture Opii Camphorata**) but in pill form; it is used to tranquilize the intestines and relieve abdominal discomfort in non-specific diarrhea.

Modern Perspective:

The effective component of this medication is the opium, which effectively relieves pain and checks diarrhea (causing constipation with chronic use). Opium in its various forms represented the only effective pain reliever available to the civil war surgeon short of anesthesia.

The camphor was felt to be helpful for so called "spasmodic" disorders, representing abrupt and recurrent events ranging from abdominal cramps to neuralgias to epilepsy. In this preparation it is probably intended to help abdominal cramping, but would not have a significant effect in that regard.

Camphor applied to the skin has a cooling and anti-itching effect.

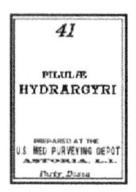

Pilulæ Hydrargyri (mercury pills; blue pills; blue mass: a mixture of elemental mercury, powdered licorice, powdered rose leaves and honey; each pill contains one grain of mercury)
Dark blue

Blue pills have similar uses to **calomel**, but it is even milder and less likely to act on the bowels in small (less than 5 grain) doses, although diarrhea may be induced. It is therefore better for chronic treatment than calomel. Doses of 2 to 5 grains each evening have a beneficial alterative effect on the inflammatory diseases, especially of the digestive organs. If no bowel movement occurs after one day a purgative should be administered. It may be combined with **opium** if an anti-inflammatory effect is desired without any purgative effect.

Modern Perspective:

The effective component of this medication is the opium, which effectively relieves pain and checks diarrhea (causing constipation with chronic use). Opium in its various forms represented the only effective pain reliever available to the civil war surgeon short of anesthesia.

The camphor was felt to be helpful for so called "spasmodic" disorders, representing abrupt and recurrent events ranging from abdominal cramps to neuralgias to epilepsy. In this preparation it is probably intended to help abdominal cramping, but would not have a significant effect in that regard.

Camphor applied to the skin has a cooling and anti-itching effect.

Period Reference:

The Elements of Materia Medica and Therapeutics – Jonathan Pereira, M.D. (Blanchard and Lee, Philadelphia, 1852) on the uses and administration of:
Mercury Pills

Preparation– The following are the directions of the British Colleges for the preparation of these pills: –

Take of Mercury one-half ounce [two *parts,* E.]; Confection of Red Roses six drachms [*three parts,* E:]; Liquorice Root, powdered., three drachms [*one part,* E.]. Rub the mercury with the confection until globules can no longer be seen; then, the liquorice being added, beat the whole together until incorporated. -[Divide the mass into five grain pills, E.] – The *Dublin College* uses the same ingredients and in the same proportion as the London College.

[The *U. S. Pharm.* orders of Mercury an ounce; Confection of Roses an ounce and a half; Liquorice Root, in powder, half an ounce. Rub the mercury with the confection until the globules disappear, then add the liquorice root, and beat the whole into a mass, to be divided into four hundred and eighty pills.]

Physiologic Effects – In full doses (as from one to fifteen grains) it frequently acts as a purgative. In small doses it is alterative, and, by repetition produces the before-mentioned constitutional effects of mercurials.

Uses – The practice of giving a blue pill at night, and a senna draught the following morning, has become somewhat popular, in consequence of its being recommended by the late Mr. Abernethy, in various disorders of the chylopoietic viscera. As an alterative, in doses of two or three grains, blue pill is frequently resorted to. Lastly, it is one of the best internal agents for exciting salivation in the various diseases for which mercury is adapted.

Administration - The usual mode of exhibiting it is in the form of pill, in the doses already mentioned; but it may also be administered when suspended in a thick mucilaginous liquid. If the object be to excite salivation, we may give five grains in the morning, and from five to ten in the evening; and to prevent purging, opium may be conjoined.

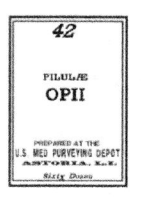

Pilulæ Opii (Opium Pills) —
White solid

This is the primary pain reliever (anodyne) in use; the effects however are complex, with primarily stimulation at low doses and narcotic effect at higher doses; as well as effects causing increased perspiration and prominent antispasmodic effects. After the main effect has passed, there is a depressed and debilitated state. At higher doses it is good for production of sleep in excitable states like delirium tremens. Due to the powerful antispasmodic effects as well as pain relief, it is indicated for tetanus, colic, urethral spasm, for quieting cough, or for tenesmus or strangury. Because of the initial stimulation, it is good for low or typhoid complaints, but should not be used in high state or inflammatory excitement.

Modern Perspective:

Opium effectively relieves pain and checks diarrhea (causing constipation with chronic use). Opium in its various forms represented the only effective pain reliever available to the civil war surgeon short of anesthesia. Morphine is still the gold standard for pain relief.

The civil war surgeon was hampered by the lack of an effective pain reliever for lesser pain. Aspirin was not widely available until the turn of the century for pain and fever relief, although

Bruce A. Evans, M.D.

folk remedies using bark preparations containing salicylates (related to aspirin) dated back to Native American use.

Period Reference:

The Elements of Materia Medica and Therapeutics – Jonathan Pereira, M.D. (Blanchard and Lee, Philadelphia, 1852) on the uses and administration of:
Opium

Uses.– Opium is undoubtedly the most important and valuable remedy of the whole Materia Medica. For other medicines we have one or more substitutes; but for opium none, at least in the large majority of cases in which its peculiar and beneficial influence is required. Its good effects are not, as is the case with some valuable medicines, remote and contingent, but they are immediate, direct, and obvious; and its operation is not attended with pain or discomfort. Farthermore, it is applied, and with the greatest success, to the relief of maladies of every day's occurrence, some of which are attended with the most acute human suffering- These circumstances, with others not necessary here to enumerate, conspire to give to opium an interest not possessed by any other article of the Materia Medica.

We employ it to fulfil various indications; some of which have been already noticed. Thus we exhibit it, under certain regulations, to rnitigate pain, to allay spasm, to promote sleep, to relieve nervous restlessness, to produce perspiration and to check profuse mucous discharges from the bronchial tubes and gastrointestinal canal. But experience has proved its value in relieving some diseases in which not one of these indications can be at all times distinctly traced.

1. *In Fevers.–* The consideration of the use of opium in fever presents peculiar difficulties. Though certain symptoms which occur in the course of this disease are, under some circumstances, most advantageously treated by opium, *yet, with* one or more of these

symptoms present, opium may, notwithstanding, be a very inappropriate remedy. The propriety or impropriety of its use, in such cases, must be determined by other circumstances, which, however, are exceedingly difficult to define and characterize. It should always be employed with great caution, giving it in small doses, and carefully watching its effects. The symptoms for which it has been resorted to are, *watchfulness, great restlessness, delirium, tremor,* and *diarrhea.* When watchfulness and great restlessness are disproportionate, from first to last, to the disorder of the vascular system, or of the constitution at large; or when these symptoms continue after excitement of the vascular system has been subdued by appropriate depletives, opium frequently proves a highly valuable remedy; nay, the safety of the patient often arises from its judicious employment. The same remarks also apply to the employment of opium for the relief of delirium; but it may be added that, in patients who have been addicted to the use of spirituous liquors, the efficacy of opium in allaying delirium is greatest. Yet I have seen opium fail to relieve the delirium of fever, even when given apparently under favourable circumstances; and I have known opium restore the consciousness of a delirious patient, and yet the case has terminated fatally. If the skin be damp, and the tongue moist, it rarely, I think, proves injurious. The absence, however, of these favourable conditions by no means precludes the employment of opium; but its efficacy is more doubtful. Dr. Holland suggests that the condition of the pupil may serve as a guide in some doubtful cases; where it is contracted, opium being contraindicated. A similar suggestion with respect to the use of belladonna was made by Dr. Graves, to which I have offered some objections. When sopor or coma supervenes in fever, the use of opium generally proves injurious. Recently, the combination of opium and emetic tartar has been strongly recommended in fever with much cerebral disturbance, by Dr. Law and Dr. Graves.

    2. *In Inflammatory Diseases.–* Opium has long been regarded as an objectionable remedy in inflammation; but it is one we frequently resort to, either for the purpose of palliating particular symptoms, or even as a powerful auxiliary antiphlogistic remedy. The statement of Dr. Young, " that opium was improper in all those diseases in which

bleeding was necessary," is, therefore, by no means correct in a very considerable number of instances. The objects for which opium is usually exhibited in inflammatory diseases are to mitigate excessive pain, to allay spasm, to relieve great restlessness, to check excessive secretion, and to act as an antiphlogistic. In employing it as an anodyne, we are to bear in mind that it is applicable to those cases only in which the pain is disproportionate to the local vascular excitement; and even then it must be employed with considerable caution; for to "stupefy the sensibility to pain, or to suspend any particular disorder of function, unless we can simultaneously lessen or remove the causes which create it, is often but to interpose a veil between our judgment and the impending danger." As an antiphlogistic, it is best given in conjunction with calomel, as recommended by Dr. R. Hamilton, of Lynn. The practice, however, does not prove equally successful in all forms of inflammation. It is best adapted for the disease when it affects membranous parts," and is much less beneficial in inflammation of the parenchymatous structure of organs. In *gastritis* and *enteritis* the use of opium has been strongly recommended by the late Dr. Armstrong. After bleeding the patient to syncope, a full opiate (as 80 or 100 drops of the tincture, or three grains of soft opium) is to be administered; and if the stomach reject it, we may give it by injection. It acts on the skin, induces quiet and refreshing sleep, and prevents what is called the hemorrhagic reaction. If the urgent symptoms return when the patient awakes, the same mode of treatment is to be followed, but combining calomel with the opium. A. third venesection is seldom required. In *peritonitis,* the same plan of treatment is to be adopted; but warm, moist applications are on no account to be omitted. Of the great value of opiates in *puerperal fever,* 'abundant evidence has been adduced by Dr. Ferguson. In *cystitis,* opium, preceded "and accompanied by bloodletting and the warm bath, is a valuable remedy; it relieves the scalding pain, by diminishing the sensibility of this viscus to the presence of the urine, and also counteracts the spasmodic contractions. In *inflammation of the walls of the pelvis of the kidney, and also of the ureters,* especially when brought on by the presence of a calculus, opium is a most valuable remedy; it diminishes the sensibility of these parts, and prevents spasm; farthermore, it relaxes the ureters, and thereby facilitates the passage of the calculus. in *inflammation of the gall-ducts,* produced by calculus, opium is likewise serviceable; but, as in the last-mentioned case, bloodletting and the warm bath should be employed simultaneously with it. In *inflammation of the mucous membranes,* attended with increased secretion, opium is a most valuable remedy. Thus, in *pulmonary catarrh,* when the first stage of the disease has passed by, and the mucous secretion is fully established, opium is frequently very beneficial; it diminishes the sensibility of the bronchial membrane to cold air, and thereby prevents cough. In severe forms of the disease, blood-letting ought to be premised. Given at the commencement of the disease, Dr. Holland says that twenty or thirty drops of laudanum will often arrest it altogether. In *diarrhea,* opium, in mild cases, is often sufficient of itself to cure the disease; it diminishes the increased muscular contractions and increased sensibility (thereby relieving pain), and at the same time checks excessive secretion. Aromatics and. chalk are advantageously combined with it. In violent cases, blood-letting should precede or accompany it. *Mild* or *English cholera,* the disease which has been so long known in this country, and which consists in irritation or inflammation of the mucous lining of the stomach, is generally most successfully treated by the use of opium; two or three doses will, in slight cases, be sufficient to effect a cure. When opium fails, the hydrocyanic acid is occasionally most effective. In *dysentery,* opium has been found very serviceable; it is best given in combination with either ipecacuanha or calomel. I have already stated that, in *inflammation, of the parenchymatous tissues of organs,* the use of opium is less frequently beneficial, but often injurious. Thus, in *inflammation of the cerebral substance,* it is highly objectionable, since it increases the determination of blood to the head, and disposes to coma. In *peripneumonia,* it is for the most part injurious; partly by its increasing the febrile symptoms, partly by its diminishing the bronchial secretion, and probably, also, by retarding the arterialization of the blood, and thereby increasing the general disorder of system. It must be admitted, however, that there are circumstances under which its use, in this disease, is justifiable. Thus, in acute peripneumonia, when bloodletting has been carried as far as the safety of the patient will admit, but without the subsidence of the disease, I have seen the repeated use of opium and calomel of essential service. Again, in the advanced stages of pneumonic inflammation, when the difficulty of breathing has abated, opium is sometimes beneficially employed to allay painful cough, and produce sleep. In *inflammation of the substance of the Liver,* opium is seldom beneficial; it checks the excretion, if not the secretion, of bile, and increases costiveness. In *rheumatic,* opium frequently evinces its happiest effects. In acute forms of the disease it is given in combination with calomel, as recommended by Dr. R. Hamilton – bloodletting being usually premised. From half a grain to two grains of opium should be given at a dose. Dr. Hope recommends gr. 7 or gr. 10 of calomel to be combined with each dose of opium. It is not necessary, or even proper, in ordinary cases, to affect the mouth by the calomel; though to this statement exceptions exist. The use of mercury may even, in some cases, be objectionable; and in such, Dover's powder will be found the best form of exhibition. This plan of treatment is well adapted for the diffuse or fibrous form of acute rheumatism; but it does not prove equally successful in the synovial forms of the disease. It is also valuable in chronic rheumatism.

8. *In Diseases of the Brain and Spinal Cord.–* In some cerebro-spinal diseases great benefit arises from the use of opium; while in other cases injury only can result from its employment. The latter effect is to be expected in inflammation of the brain, and in apoplectic cases. In other words, in those cerebral maladies obviously connected with, or dependent on, an excited condition of the vascular system of the brain, opium acts injuriously. Rut there are many disordered conditions of the cerebro-spinal functions, the intensity of which bears no proportion to that of the derangement of the vascular system of the brain; and there are other deviations from the healthy functions in which no change in the cerebral circulation can be detected. In these cases, opium or morphia frequently evinces its best effects. In *insanity,* its value has been properly insisted on by Dr. Seymour. He, as well as Messrs. Reverley and Phillips, employed the acetate of morphia. Its good effects were manifested rather in the low,

desponding, or melancholic forms of the disease, than in the excited conditions; though I have seen great relief obtained in the latter form of the disease by full doses. Opium is sometimes employed by drunkards to relieve *intoxication.* I knew a medical man addicted to drinking, and who, for many years, was accustomed to take a large dose of laudanum whenever he was intoxicated. and was called to see a patient. On one occasion, being more than ordinarily inebriated, he swallowed an excessive dose of laudanum, and died in a few hours of apoplexy.

In *delirium tremens,* the efficacy of opium is almost universally admitted. Its effects, however, require to be carefully watched; for large doses of it, frequently repeated; sometimes hasten coma and other bad symptoms. If there be much fever, or evident marks of determination of blood to the head, it should be used with great caution, and ought to be preceded by loss of blood, cold applications to the head, and other antiphlogistic measures. Though opium is to be looked on as a chief remedy in this disease, yet it is not to be regarded as a specific. Dr. Law speaks in high terms of its association with emetic tartar. I have before noticed the use of opium in alleviating some of the *cerebral symptoms which occur during fever.*

In *spasmodic and convulsive diseases* opium is a most important remedy. In *local spasms produced by topical irritants,* it is a most valuable agent, as I have already stated; for example, *in spasm of the gall-ducts* or *of the ureters,* brought on by the presence of calculi; in colic, and in *painful spasmodic contractions of the bladder,* or *rectum,* or *uterus.* In *spasmodic stricture* opium is sometimes useful. In genuine *spasmodic asthma,* which probably depends on a spasmodic condition of the muscular fibres investing the bronchial tubes, a full dose of opium generally gives temporary relief; but the recurrence of the paroxysms is seldom influenced by opium. There are several reasons for believing that one effect of narcotics in dyspnea is to diminish the necessity for respiration. Laennec states that when given to relieve the extreme dyspnea of mucous catarrh, it frequently produces a speedy but temporary cessation of the disease; and if we explore the respiration by the stethoscope, we find it the same as during the paroxysm – a proof that the benefit obtained consists simply in a diminution of the necessity for respiration. That the necessities of the system for atmospheric air vary at different periods, and from different circumstances, is sufficiently established by the experiments of Dr. Prout, and it appears that they are diminished during sleep, at which time, according to Dr. Edwards, the transpiration is increased. Moreover, the phenomena of hybernating animals also bear on this point; for during their state of torpidity, or hybernation, their respiration is proportionally diminished.

In the *convulsive diseases (chorea, epilepsy,* and *tetanus)* opium has been used, with variable success; in fact, the conditions of system under which these affections occur, may be, at different times, of an opposite nature; so that a remedy which is proper in one case is often improper in another. In *tetanus,* opium was at one time a favourite remedy, and is undoubtedly at times a remedy of considerable value. But it is remarkable that the susceptibility of the system to its influence is greatly diminished during tetanus. I have already referred to the enormous quantities which may, at this time, be taken with impunity. In 128 cases noticed by Mr. Curling, opium in various forms, and in conjunction with other remedies, was employed in 84 cases; and of these, 45 recovered. Notwithstanding, however, the confidence of the profession in its efficacy is greatly diminished.

Lastly, opium occasionally proves serviceable in several forms of *headache,* especially after loss of blood. I have seen it give great relief in some cases of what are commonly termed nervous headaches; while in others, with apparently the same indications, it has proved injurious. Chomel applied, with good effect, opium cerate to a blistered surface of the scalp, to relieve headache.

4. *In Diseases of the Chest.*– In some affections of the heart and of the organs of respiration opium is beneficial. I have already alluded to its employment in *catarrh, peripnenmonia,* and *spasmodic asthma.* In the first of these maladies caution is often requisite in its use. "In an aged person, for example, suffering under *chronic bronchitis* or *catarrhal influenza* – and gasping, it may be, under the difficulties of cough and expectoration – an opiate, by suspending these very

struggles, may become the cause of danger and death. The effort here is needed for the recovery of free respiration; and if suppressed too long, mucus accumulates in the bronchial cells, its extrication thence becomes impossible, and breathing ceases altogether."

5. *In Maladies of the Digestive Organs* – I have already referred to the use of opium in *gastritis, enteritis, peritonitis, diarrhea, dysentery, colic, the passage of gall-stones,* and in *hepatitis.* With respect to the use of opium *in hepatic affections,* I am disposed to think, with Dr. Holland, that, with the exception of the painful passage of a gall-stone through the ducts, there is scarcely a complaint of the liver and its appendages "where opium may not be said to be hurtful, though occasionally and indirectly useful when combined with other.means." *In poisoning by acrid substances* opium is used with advantage to lessen the susceptibility of the alimentary canal, and thereby to diminish the violence of the operation of these local irritants. Cantharides, all the drastic purgatives, when taken in excessive doses (as elaterium, colocynth, gamboge, scamrnony, and craton oil or seeds), and Arum *maculatum,* may be mentioned as examples of the substances alluded to. Besides the above-mentioned beneficial operation, opium allays the spasmodic contractions of *the* bowels, relieves pain, and checks inordinate secretion and exhalation.

In poisoning by corrosives (the strong mineral acids and alkalies, for example), opium diminishes the sensibility of the alimentary canal; it cannot, of course, alter the chemical influence of the poisons, but it may prove useful by allaying the consequences of inflammation.

As meconic acid is said to be an antidote in cases of poisoning by corrosive sublimate, opium, in full doses, may perhaps be administered with some advantage when other antidotes cannot be procured.

In poisoning by the preparations of arsenic, of lead, and of copper, opium is sometimes found useful.

6. *In maladies of the urino-genital apparatus* opium is a most valuable remedy. It mitigates pain, allays spasmodic action, checks copious mucous secretion, and diminishes irritation. Its use for one or

more of these purposes in *nephritis, cystitis, the passage of urinary calculi,* and *spasmodic stricture,* has been already pointed *out. In irritable bladder* it is an invaluable remedy, especially in conjunction with liquor potassae. *In irritation* and *various painful affections of the uterus,* and in *chordee,* the value of opium is well known. In the treatment of the *phosphatic diathesis* it is the only remedy that can be employed, according to Dr. Prout, to diminish the unnatural irritability of the system.

Of all remedies for that hitherto intractable malady, *diabetes,* opium has been found to give the most relief. Under its use the specific gravity, saccharine quality, and quantity of urine have been diminished. It has not, however, hitherto succeeded in permanently curing this disease. Dr. Prout has also found it serviceable when there is an excess *of urea in the urine.*

7. As an Anodyne.— To relieve pain by dulling the sensibility of the body, opium is, of all substances, the most useful, and the most to be relied on for internal exhibition. We sometimes use it to alleviate the pain of inflammation, as already mentioned; to diminish spasm and the sensibility of the part in calculi of the gall-ducts, in the ureters, and even when in the urinary bladder; to relieve pain in the various forms of scirrhus and carcinoma, in which diseases opium is our sheet-anchor; to allay the pain arising from the presence of foreign bodies in wounds; to prevent or relieve after-pains; to diminish the pain of menstruation; and, lastly, as an anodyne in neuralgia. As a *benember* or *topical anodyne* it is greatly inferior to aconite. Hence, in neuralgia, the latter is much more successful than opium. (See *Aconitum.)*

8. In Hemorrhages.— Opium is at times serviceable to obviate certain *ill effects of hemorrhages;* as when there is great irritability attended with a small and frequent pulse, and also to relieve that painful throbbing about the head so often observed after large evacuations of blood. In or immediately after *uterine hemorrhage* the use of opium has been objected to, on the ground that it might prevent the contraction of the womb; but where the employment of opium is otherwise indicated, this theoretical objection deserved no weight. In *bronchial hemorrhage* it is at times a valuable remedy, and may be associated with acetate of lead (notwithstanding the chemical objections to the mixture) with good effect.

9. *In Mortification.–* When mortification is attended with excessive pain, opium is resorted to. In that kind of mortification called *gangrene senilis,* which commences without any visible cause, by a small purple spot on the toes, heels, or other parts of the extremities, and which sometimes arises from an ossified condition of the arteries, Mr. Pott strongly recommended opium, in conjunction with a stimulating plan of treatment, and experience has fully proved its great efficacy.

10. *In Venereal Diseases.–* Opium is frequently employed in venereal diseases to prevent the action of mercurials on the bowels during salivation; also to allay the pain of certain venereal sores, and venereal diseases of the bones. By some it has, in addition, been employed as an anti-venereal remedy; and, according to Michaelis and others, with success. Moreover, it is stated by Dr. Ananian, who practised at Constantinople, that those persons who were in the habit of taking opium rarely contracted the venereal disease. But opium possesses no specific anti-venereal powers. It has appeared to me, on several occasions, to promote the healing of venereal sores.

11. In various forms of *ulcers,* and in *granulating wounds* the efficacy of opium has been satisfactorily established by Mr. Skey. Richter and others had already noticed its good effects; but their statements had attracted little attention. Mr. Grant, in 1785, pointed out the efficacy of opium in the treatment of foul ulcers, attended with a bad discharge, and much pain. He ascribed these symptoms to "morbid irritability," which the opium removed. Its use is prejudicial in ulcers attended with inflammation, in the florid or sanguineous temperament, and in childhood. But in the chronic or callous ulcer, in the so-called varicose ulcer, in recent ulcers (from wounds), in which granulation proceeds slowly, or in other cases, the efficacy of opium, administered in small doses (as ten drops of laudanum three times daily), is most manifest, especially in elderly persons, and in those whose constitutions have been debilitated by disease, labour,

spirituous liquors, &c. It appears to promote the most genial warmth, to give energy to the extreme arteries, and thereby to maintain an equal balance of the circulation throughout every part of the body, and to animate the dormant energies of healthy action.

12. The *external application* of opium is comparatively but little resorted to, and for two reasons: in the first place, its topical effects are slight; and secondly, its specific effects on the brain and general system are not readily produced through the skin. Aconite and belladonna greatly exceed opium in their topical effects. The following are some of the local uses of opium: In *ophthalmia,* the wine of opium is dropped into the eye when there is excessive pain (see *Vinum Opia).* In *painful and foul sores,* opiates are used with occasional good effects. Mr. Grant applied the tincture twice a day, in an oatmeal poultice, to irritable sores. Opiate *frictions* have been employed as topical anodynes, and to affect. the general system. - Thus, in *chronic rheumatism and sprains,* the opium liniment proves a useful application. In *maniacal delirium,* as well as some other cerebral disorders, Mr. Ward employed, with apparently beneficial effects, opiate frictions; for example, one-half ounce of opium, mixed with gr. 4 of camphor, 4 scruples of lard, and one drachm of olive oil. In *neuralgic affections,* an opiate cerate, or finely powdered hydrochlorate of morphia, applied to a blistered surface, occasionally gives relief. In *gastrodynia,* it may be applied in the same way to the epigastrium (Holland). In *gonorrhea and gleet,* opium injections have been used. In *spasmodic stricture, diseases of the prostate gland,* and in g*onorrhoea to prevent chordee,* an opiate suppository is a useful form of employing opium, especially where it is apt to disagree with the stomach. In *nervous and spasmodic affections* (as some forms of asthma), the endermic application of opium or morphia, applied along the course of the spine, is often singularly beneficial, when all methods of depletion and counter-irritation have proved utterly unavailing (Holland). In *toothache,* opium is applied to the hollow of a carious tooth. Dr. Row speaks in the highest terms of the efficacy of the external application of opium *in inflammatory diseases,* but especially *bronchitis* and *croup.*

Administration.– Opium is given, *in substance,* in the form of pill, powder, lozenge, or electuary. The dose is subject to great variation, depending on the age and habits of the patient, the nature of the disease, and the particular object for which we wish to employ it. In a general way, we consider from an eighth of a grain to half a grain a *small dose* for an adult. We give it to this extent in persons unaccustomed to its use, when we require its stimulant effects, and in mild catarrhs and diarrhoeas. From half a grain to two grains we term a *medium dose,* and employ it in this quantity as an ordinary anodyne and soporific. From two to five grains we denominate a *full* or *large dose,* and give it to relieve excessive pain, violent spasm, in some inflammatory diseases after bloodletting, in tetanus, &c. These are by no means to be regarded as the limits of the use of opium. *Opium pills (pilulae opii)* may be prepared either with crude or powdered opium. The latter has the advantage of a more speedy operation, in consequence of its more ready solution in the gastric liquor. Employed as a *suppository,* opium is used in larger doses than when given by the stomach. Five grains, made into a cylindric mass with soap, may be introduced into the rectum, to allay irritation in the urinogenital organs.

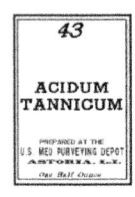

Acidum Tannicum (tannic acid) -
White or slightly yellow powder

This is a vegetable astringent (drying and tissue tightening agent) without the tonic effects of the mineral astringents such as the iron compounds. Because of this it is better for use in active hemorrhage from the bowels than agents which might be expected to stimulate the circulation. It is active in a small dose (2-5 grains in water) so irritates the bowel less than some others, making it preferable in diarrhea.

Modern Perspective:

Tannic acid is a drying agent used externally, and does have the effect of retarding bleeding - it is a component, along with alum, of many styptic pencils.

Extrapolating from this, 19th century physicians assumed that it would have a beneficial "drying" effect on internal tissues, helping with diarrhea and dysentery and internal hemorrhage, but it has no such effect.

Very large doses can cause stomach inflammation, fatal liver damage, and kidney damage.

Period Reference:

The Elements of Materia Medica and Therapeutics – Jonathan Pereira, M.D. (Blanchard and Lee, Philadelphia, 1852) on the uses and administration of:
Tannic Acid

Considered as a medicine, tannic acid is a powerful agent of the astringent class. As a *topical* remedy it is probably the most powerful of all vegetable astringents or styptics. Its chemical action on fibrine, albumen, and gelatin explains this. It is the active principle of a very large proportion of vegetable astringents (see vol. i.; pp. 200 and 248). Given to a dog in doses of from 7 and one-half grains to about 93 grains, it did not affect the health of the animal: it caused constipation, but its appetite remained the same. The urine gradually became darker coloured and opake, and. was found to contain both gallic and pyrogallic acids and humus-like substances. The tannic acid had become converted into these bodies in its passage through the animal system. The gallic acid was detected by the blackish blue precipitate produced by the persalts of iron, and by no precipitate being produced with gelatin. Pyrogallic acid was detected by the bluish black precipitate produced. by the proto-salts of iron. On the human subject tannic acid also operates as a constipating agent when given in a sufficient dose and frequently repeated; Cavarra states that 2.5 grains taken three days successively produced this effect on himself. The *remote* effects of tannic acid are not so obvious, but they appear to be astringent, though in a much feebler degree. As the tannic acid becomes changed into gallic acid in its passage through the system, it is probably the latter agent which operates on remote parts as an astringent when tannic acid is administered. If this opinion be correct., tannic acid would act, as Dr. Garron has suggested, less powerfully as a remote astringent than an equal weight of gallic acid. But, as a topical astringent, tannic is far more powerful than gallic acid; because its chemical reaction on albumen, gelatin, and fibrine is more energetic.

Tannic acid is used as an astringent chiefly in hemorrhages and profuse secretions; and also to constringe relaxed fibres. In hemorrhages, it has been used both topically, as a styptic (in bleeding gums, piles, and uterine hemorrhage), and remotely, as an astringent (in hemorrhage from the lungs, stomach, bowels, kidneys, and uterus). In chronic fluxes it has likewise been employed both as a topical and a remote remedy: topically in gonorrhoea, gleet, leucorrhoea, and. ophthalmia; remotely in pulmonary catarrh, diarrhoea, dysentery, leucorrhoea, gonorrhoea, and. cystirrhoea. To restrain the phthisical sweating it has been recommended by Charvet and others, and Giadorow states that, given in combination with opium, he cured. (?) two cases of diabetes by it. To constringe fibres, it is applied. to spongy gums and prolapsed bowel. As an application to sores, it has been employed by Ricord in chancres, and by Mr. Druitt in sore nipples. Dr. Scott Alison has recently recommended its use in various other cases: as a tonic or peptic in dyspepsia; as an "histogenetic" to promote the genesis and improve the quality of the blood, in rickets, &c.; as a nervine in nervous debility and languor; and to arrest or retard the growth of heterologous formations (tubercle, malignant disease, &c.). It has likewise been given as an antidote to check excessive vomiting from ipecacuanha or emetina.– Tannic acid may be administered in doses of from 8 to 10 or more grains, in powder, pill, or solution. When we employ it as a remote agent, the pill-form seems to be the most appropriate mode of exhibition.– As a lotion or injection, it may be used in the form of aqueous solution containing from 4 to 6 or more grains in the fluidounce. It has also been employed in the form of ointment composed of 2 drachms of the acid dissolved in two fluiddrachms of distilled water and mixed with 12 ounces of lard.

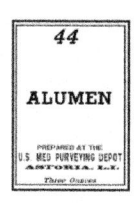

Alumen (alum) -
White, efflorescent salt

Alum may be used internally as astringent (drying and tightening agent) in passive hemorrhage, chronic dysentery, and diarrheas. Topical use includes as a gargle for mouth lesions including mercury induced lesions. Finely powdered alum may be used as a styptic, but it is less efficient than **Liquor Ferri Persuphatus**

Modern Perspective:

Alum is a drying agent used externally, and does have the effect of retarding bleeding - it is a component, along with tannic acid, of many styptic pencils.

Extrapolating from this, 19th century physicians assumed that it would have a beneficial "drying" effect on internal tissues, helping with diarrhea and dysentery and internal hemorrhage, but it has no such effect.

Toxicity internally is minimal and consists mainly of irritation due to production of sulfuric acid from hydrolysis of the salt.

Period Reference:

The Elements of Materia Medica and Therapeutics – Jonathan Pereira, M.D. (Blanchard and Lee, Philadelphia, 1852) on the uses and administration of:**Alum**

Uses – Alum is employed both as an external or topical, and as an internal remedy.

a. As a topical remedy.– Solutions of alum are sometimes employed *to produce contraction or corrugation of the tissues,* and. thereby to prevent displacement of parts, especially when accompanied with excessive secretion. Thus if, is used as a gargle in relaxation of the uvula with evident advantage. In the early stage of prolapsus of the rectum, a solution of alum, applied as a wash, is sometimes of service, especially when the disease occurs in infants. Washes or injections containing alum are of occasional benefit in prolapsus of the uterus.

In hemorrhages, whether proceeding from an exhalation or exudation from the extremities or pores of the minute vessels, or from the rupture of a bloodvessel, a solution, or, in some cases, the powder of alum, may be used with advantage as a *styptic,* to constringe the capillary vessels, and close their bleeding orifices. Thus in epistaxis, when it is considered advisable to arrest the hemorrhage, assistance may be gained by the injection of alum into the nostrils, or by the introduction of lint moistened with the solution. Where this fails to give relief, Finely-powdered, alum may be employed in the manner of snuff. In hemorrhage from the mouth or throat, gargles containing alum are useful. In haematemesis, as well as in intestinal hemorrhage, alum whey may be administered; though, of course, no reliance can be placed on it, as the hemorrhage usually depends on circumstances which astringents merely cannot be expected to obviate. In uterine hemorrhage, a sponge soaked in a solution of alum may be introduced into the vagina with good. effect. To check the hemorrhoidal flux when immoderate, washes or enemata containing alum may be employed. To stop the bleeding after leech-bites in children, a saturated solution, or the powder of alum, may be applied to the punctures.

In certain inflammations, alum has been used as a *repellent* (see *ante,* p. 201); that is, it has been applied to the inflamed part in order to produce contraction of the distended. vessels, and thereby to diminish the quantity of blood in the seat of the disease in a manner almost mechanical. Thus in the first stage of ophthalmia it is sometimes considered expedient to cut short the disease by the application of a strong astringent solution (as a saturated solution of alum or of acetate of lead). " It is not to be denied," observes Dr. Jacob, " that such applications may have the effect of arresting the progress of the disease at once; but if they have not that effect, they are liable to produce an increase of irritation." But, as the details necessary for making the student acquainted with all the circumstances respecting the use of stimulating or astringent applications in the first stage of ophthalmia are too lengthened and numerous to admit of their proper discussion in this work, I must refer for further particulars to the essay of Dr. Jacob before quoted, as well as to the treatises of writers on ophthalmic surgery. I may, however, add, that whatever difference of opinion exists as to the propriety of these applications in the first stage of ophthalmia, all are agreed as to their value after the violence of vascular action has been subdued. In the treatment of the purulent ophthalmia of infants, no remedy is perhaps equal to an alum wash.

In angina membranacea, called by Bretanneau diphtheritis, great importance has been attached. to the employment of local applications. Of these, hydrochloric acid, calomel, and alum, have, in succession, been highly praised by this writer. In order to promote the expulsion of the false membrane, he recommends the insufflation of finely-powdered alum. This is effected by placing a drachm of it in a tube, and blowing it into the throat. Velpeau has subsequently confirmed the statements of Bretonneau, and extended the use of alum to other inflammatory affections of the throat, as those arising in scarlatina, small-pox, &c. In these cases powdered alum may be applied to the affected. parts by means of the index finger. Gargles containing this salt will be found useful in most kinds of sore-throat, ulcerations of the mouth and gums, aphthae, &c. In inflammation of the uvula, accompanied with membraniform exudation, alum washes are serviceable both in children and adults.

Alum has been employed as an *astringent,* to diminish or stop excessive secretion from the mucous surfaces. Thus a weak solution of this salt is used to repress the discharge in the latter stages of conjunctival inflammation; to check profuse ptya- lism, whether from the use of mercury or other causes; and to remove gleet or leucorrhoea. In old-standing diarrhoeas, it has been administered, in combination with the vegetable astringents (kino, for example), with occasional ad.vantage. It is also applied to check profuse secretion from ulcers.

b. As *an internal remedy.–* Alum has been employed, in conjunction with nutmeg, as a remedy for intermittents. Given just before the expected paroxysm, it has, in some cases,. prevented it. In the treatment of *lead colic,* alum has been found more successful than any other agent or class of remedies. It was first used in this disease by a Dutch physician, named Grashuis, and was afterwards administered in fifteen cases by Dr. Percival with great success. Its efficacy has been fully established by Kapeler (physician to the Hopital St. Antoine, in Paris) and Gendrin, and by Dr. Copland, as well as by several other distinguishecl authorities. It allays vomiting, abates flatulence, mitigates pain, and opens the bowels more certainly than any other medicine, and frequently when other powerful remedies have failed. It should be given in full doses (as from a scruple to two drachms), dissolved in some demulcent liquid. (as gum-water) every three or four hours. Opium and (according to Dr. Copland) camphor may be advantageously conjoined. Kapeler also employs oleaginous enemata. The modus operandi of alum in lead colic is not very clear. The benefit has been ascribed by some to the chemical action of the sulphuric acid on the lead, contained in the intestines; and in support of this view must be mentioned the fact, that other sulphates (as those of magnesia, soda, zinc, and copper), as well as free sulphuric acid, have been successfully employed in lead colic. But, on the other hand, the presence of lead in the primae viae or evacuations, and, consequently, the formation of sulphate of lead in saturnine colic, have not been demonstrated; though the experiments of Dr. C. G Mitscherlich have shown that, when the acetate of lead is swallowed, the greater part of it forms an insoluble combination with the gastro-intestinal mucus, and in this state may remain some time in the alimentary canal. Moreover, alum has been found successful by

Kopp in other varieties of colic not caused by lead, and unaccompanied by constipation. Dr. Copland is disposed. to ascribe the benefit of alum and. other sulphates in lead colic to their "exciting the action of the partially-paralyzed muscular coat of the bowels, arid. thereby enabling them to expel retained matters of a morbid or noxious description" – an explanation which is inconsistent with the observation of Kopp just quoted.

Alum is administered internally in several other diseases, of which a brief notice only can be given. In passive or asthenic hemorrhages from distant organs; as haemoptysis, menorrhagia and other uterine hemorrhages, haematuria, &c. In colliquative sweating, diabetes, gleet, gonorrhoea, and leucorrhoea. In the three latter diseases it may be combined with cubebs. Kreysig has advised its use in dilatation of the heart and aortic aneurism. More recently, Dzondi has also recommended it in these diseases; and. Sundelin has mentioned a case of supposed dilatation of the heart, in which relief was gained by the use of alum. In chronic diarrhea, alum is occasionally serviceable.

Administration.– The dose of alum is from ten grains to one or two scruples. It may be taken in the form of powder, or made into pills with some tonic extract, or in solution. To prevent nausea, an aromatic (as nutmeg) should be conjoined. A pleasant mode of exhibition is in the form of *alum whey (serum aluminosum,* seu *serum lactis aluminatum),* prepared by boiling two drachms of powdered alum with a pint of milk, then straining: the dose is a wineglassful. The *saccharum aluminatum* of the Prussian Pharmacopoeia is composed of equal parts of white sugar and alum: it may be given to children as well as adults. In prescribing alum, it is to be remembered that the vegetable astringents decompose it; by which the astringent property of the mixture is probably diminished.

For topical uses, alum is used in the form of powder, solution, and poultice. Powder of crystallized alum is applied to the mouth and throat as before mentioned. Solutions of alum are made, for topical purposes, of various strengths, according to the. object in view.

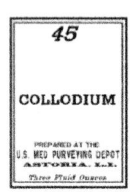

Collodium (etheral solution of gun cotton; Maynard's adhesive liquid) -
Transparent liquid

The main use is as an adhesive for wound edges and as a dressing covering ulcers. Linen squares may be placed over a wound extending to sound skin on either side, where the collodium may be placed by application with a hair pencil as an adhesive, to bring the sides of the wound into opposition. It may be painted directly over a small wound or ulcer as protectant.

Period Reference:

From A Manual of Minor Surgery by John H.r Packard, M.D., 1863

COLLODION, made by dissolving gun-cotton in sulphuric ether, is much used as an adhesive material. After operations on the eye, it is employed to keep the lid closed. For this purpose, or for keeping the lips of a wound in apposition, a piece of fine soft rag is laid with its centre directly over the affected part, and then the collodion is painted on with a camel's-hair pencil, so as to attach each end of the rag to the sound. skin beneath it. Thus the wound or the eye is left free from irritation, or may have any other suitable dressing confined, upon it. Small wounds may be simply painted over with the *collodion,* which is also supplied in some cases for the sake of the contraction undergone by it in drying; small naevi may sometimes be entirely discussed in. this way, and occasionally even vascular engorgements of the testicle, breast and other organs.

Mr. Hubbell, the well-known druggist of this city, prepares a non-contractile form of collodion, by adding to every glass of liquid Venice turpentine or of castor oil. The former makes a better preparation, unless it

is specially desirable to avoid irritating the parts. Zither will be found to possess advantages over collodion as commonly prepared.

An excellent substitute for blisters of the ordinary form is obtained by dissolving an ethereal extract of cantharides in collodion. It is called *blistering* or *cantharidal collodion;* the mode of employing it being simply to paint it over the desired extent of surface by means of a camel's-hair pencil. Its action is hastened by laying over it a piece of oiled silk, so as to prevent the evaporation of the ether. Some surgeons also use collodion as a vehicle for the application of creosote, in cases of erysipelas or erythema of the traumatic variety.

Whenever it is desirable to remove collodion, either simple or medicated, this may readily be done by dissolving it away with ether.

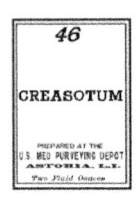

Creasotum (Creosote) -
Colorless, oleaginous liquid

This is used externally to promote healing of wounds, eruptions, and especially scaly eruptions. It may be added to warm water dressings as a deodorant. Put 50 drops in a pint of water to be used as a daily wash for a wound showing a sloughing tendency.

Modern Perspective:

This substance does have some deodorizing properties when applied to "mortifying" wounds.

It was also felt to have disinfectant properties, although the understanding of that term was different than the current implication of preventing bacterial infection. Disinfectants were applied to inflamed wounds to retard "mortification" - the progression to tissue death associated with the sloughing off of dead tissue and "fetid" smells. The concept of applying disinfectants prior to inflammatory change - what we would recognize as infection - to prevent that occurance was unknown until Lister publicized the use of such a substance - phenolic or carbolic acid - for just that purpose, and revolutionized the practice of surgery.

Interestingly, the British form of creosote, derived from oil, contained substantial amounts of carbolic (phenolic) acid, and would have been a much more effective disinfectant (in the modern sense) than the American product which - derived from wood products - did not.

This substance likely did benefit proliferative, scaling skin disorders such as psoriasis.

Period Reference:

The Elements of Materia Medica and Therapeutics – Jonathan Pereira, M.D. (Blanchard and Lee, Philadelphia, 1852) on the uses and administration of:
Creasote

Uses.–As an *external* agent, creasote may frequently be employed with great advantage. It has been successfully applied to relieve *toothache*. After carefully cleaning out the cavity of the tooth, a drop of creasote, or an *alcoholic solution* of this principle, may be introduced by means of a camel's hair pencil, and the cavity filled with cotton soaked in this liquid. As a local application to chronic skin diseases (particularly the different forms of porrigo, impetigo, eczema) it is of considerable value. Where a caustic application is required, it may be applied undiluted; but for other purposes, it is used either in the form of ointment, or dissolved in water as a wash. Creasote may be beneficially used as an application to foul and indolent ulcers. It serves the double purpose of stimulating the living surface (and thereby of changing the quality of actions going on in the part), and also of preventing the putrefaction of the secreted matters. It is sometimes applied pure, but more commonly diluted with water. Lupus is said to have healed under the employment of an ointment of creasote. In hemorrhages creasote acts as a most efficient styptic, partly in consequence of its power of coagulating albuminous liquids, and thereby of causing the formation of a clot, and partly by causing contraction of the bleeding vessels. *Creasote water* (prepared by mixing one part of creasote with eighty parts of water) may be applied either to bleeding wounds and leech-bites, or introduced into the vagina in uterine hemorrhage, by means of pledgets of lint soaked in it. There are many other purposes for which creasote has been applied as a local agent, but which I think it sufficient merely to name, referring the reader to the various papers and works before quoted for farther information. It has been employed to check caries, to restrain excessive suppuration, and to repress fungous granulations in burns and scalds; to act as a counter-irritant in chronic ophthalmia, in which disease it is sometimes dropped into the eye on the same principle that nitrate of silver and other local stimulants are used; and to remove condylomatous and other excrescences. The inhalation of creasote vapour is occasionally useful in relieving excessive bronchial secretion. Dr. Elliotson cured two cases of glanders in the human subject by injecting an aqueous solution of creasote up the affected nostril.

Administration.– Creasote may be given, at the commencement of its use, in doses of one or two drops diffused through an ounce of some aromatic water by the aid of mucilage: the dose should be gradually increased. As before mentions, in one case forty drops were given with impunity; in another instance, ninety drops were administered in less than half a day without any bad symptom.
As a caustic, undiluted creasote is sometimes applied by means of a camel-hair pencil.

Lotions, gargles, or injections of creasote are prepared by dissolving from two to six drops (according to the circumstances of each case) in an ounce of water. A solution of this kind is sometimes mixed with poultices.
The inhalation of creasote vapour may be effected by diffusing a few drops of creasote through water or a mucilaginous liquid, and breathing through this by means of the ordinary inhaling bottle.

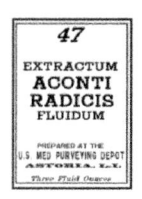

Extractum Aconti Radicis Fluidum (fluid extract of aconite root) -
Yellowish-brown liquid

(Use has been documented since 1762)

This medicine causes decreased force and frequency of the pulse. It is used in doses of ½ - 2 grains, morning and night, and as a sedative for reducing the force of the circulation in sthenic disorders such as high fevers, acute rheumatism, neuralgia, and epilepsy.

Modern Perspective:

This is a significant poison, and 20-40 ml. of a 10% tincture may be fatal (2-4 grams = 30-60 grains). The fatal effects begin with warmth and tingling on mucous membranes, followed by various central nervous system effects such as nausea, vomiting, diarrhea, incoordination, dizziness, slowed breathing and convulsions as well as direct effects on the heart.

These later depressant effects on the heart were precisely the goal of its medical use, since the abnormal excitement of the pounding, rapid pulse of inflammatory diseases could be damped down by such action, moving the patient closer to the "normal state". Unfortunately, such treatment did not benefit the patient since in most cases these circulation symptoms are physiologic and compensatory. The effect may be similar, if less offensive, than bleeding for the same disease.

Period Reference:

The Elements of Materia Medica and Therapeutics – Jonathan Pereira, M.D. (Blanchard and Lee, Philadelphia, 1852) on the uses and administration of:
Aconite

Uses – A. knowledge of the physiological effects of aconite suggests the therapeutical uses of this medicine. A benumber is obviously the physiological remedy for increased sensibility (pain) of the nerves. As a *topical remedy,* aconite is most valuable for the relief of neuralgic and rheumatic pains. In *neuralgia,* no remedy, I believe, will be found equal to it. One application of the tincture produces some amelioration, and, after a few times' use, it frequently happens that the patient is cured. In some cases the benefit seems almost magical. In others, however, the remedy entirely fails to give any permanent relief. Though the pathology of this disease be but little understood, yet we know that the causes of it, and the conditions under which it occurs, are by no means uniform. We are, therefore, easily prepared to believe that while in some cases aconite may prove beneficial, in others it may be useless. I do not think that, in any it proves injurious. The causes of neuralgia are, however, usually obscure, and therefore we are in most cases not able to determine *a priori* the probability or the reverse of the beneficial agency of aconite. Hence its employment must be, for the most part, empirical. I have observed that, when it succeeds, it gives more or less relief at the first application. When the disease depends on inflammation, aconite will be found, I think, an unavailing remedy. In a painful affection of the nerves of the face, arising from inflammation of the socket of a tooth, it gave no relief. In *rheumatic pains,* unaccompanied with local swelling or redness, aconite is frequently of great service. In painful conditions of the intercostal and other respiratory muscles, occurring in rheumatic individuals, I have found this remedy most valuable. In one case of *sciatica* it gave partial relief; but in most cases in which I have tried it, it has failed. In *lumbago,* I have not tried it. Dr. Turnbull states that a lady was cured of this disease by the aconite ointment. In *acute rheumatism,* its application has not proved successful in my hands; but I have been informed of cases occurring to others in which it has been of great service.

Aconite has been administered *internally* in various diseases, principally on the recommendation of Storck. It has been employed as a narcotic (anodyne) sedative, sudorific, resolvent, and diuretic. The diseases in which it has been employed are *rheumatism, gout, scrofula, phthisis, syphilis, some skin disegses, scirrhus* and *cancer, intermittents, dropsies, paralysis, epilepsy, amaurosis, uterine affections,* and *hypertrophy of the heart.* In the large majority of these maladies scarcely any practitioner now believes in its efficacy. Fouquier gave it very extensive trials without obtaining much relief from it, except as a diuretic in *passive dropsies.* In *rheumatism,* it has frequently proved serviceable when combined with a sudorific regimen. I have seen it give great relief in rheumatic pains. In *hypertrophy of the heart* it has been recommended by Dr. Lombard on account of its decidedly sedative effects.

Administration.– The only preparations of aconite, whose activity may be relied on, are the *tincture* of the root (made with rectified spirit), the *alcoholic ex*tract, and Morson's *aconitina.* The *powder* is given in doses of one or two grains, gradually increased, until some effects are produced; but no reliance can be placed on it. When of good quality, it causes numbness and tingling of the lips and tongue a few minutes after its application to these parts.

Antidotes– See the treatment for poisoning by tobacco. In Mr. Sherwen's case great benefit was obtained by the abstraction of ten ounces of blood from the jugular vein.

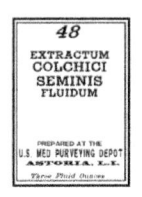

Extractum Colchici Seminis Fluidum (fluid extract of colchicum seed) -
Reddish-brown liquid

(Use has been documented since 1763)

    This medication provides pain relief and sedation without any effect on secretions, and is especially useful in gout and to a lesser extent rheumatism, unaccompanied by fever, hot, dry skin, or other signs of general excitement of the system. Its beneficial action in gout is remarkable. It is used in doses of 1-2 grains 2 to 3 times per day. Its use in sthenic diseases generally is limited by distressing nausea, and occasionally vomiting and purging, so alternative treatments are preferred.

Modern Perspective:

    This substance is one of the truly effective medications of the era, but only when used for gout. Colchicine has a direct effect on the process of inflammation and a further, more specific, curative effect on the acute inflammation of gout.

    It is, in fact, still used in acute attacks of gouty arthritis. Its use in other kinds of inflammation, with a few unusual exceptions, has been taken by much less toxic medications such as aspirin, ibuprofen, and other non-steroidal anti-inflammatory drugs (NSAIDs).

In the 1860s, the benefit to gout was well known, as was the lesser benefit to other inflammatory diseases such as arthritis of other causes. From a modern point of view, this was a medication with one very effective use, and other uses of less, but still definite, benefit.

More than 3 mg. of the PURE alkaloid (the corresponding concentration of which in this preparation is unknown) may cause death following throat burning, nausea, diarrhea, abdominal pain, kidney failure, delirium, convulsions, respiratory failure, coma, and circulatory collapse. Some of these symptoms limit chronic use of smaller doses to prevent gout, and can be very dangerous if the drug is not immediately discontinued.

Period Reference:

The Elements of Materia Medica and Therapeutics – Jonathan Pereira, M.D. (Blanchard and Lee, Philadelphia, 1852) on the uses and administration of:
Uses -

1. *In Gout.*– The circumstances which of late years have led to the extensive employment of colchicum in gout are the following: About seventy years ago, M. Husson, a military officer in the service of the king of France, discovered, as he informs us, a plant possessed of extraordinary virtues in the cure of various diseases. From this plant he prepared a remedy called *Eau Medicinale,* which acquired great celebrity for abating the pain and cutting short the paroxysms of gout. Various attempts were made to discover the nature of its active principle. In 1782, MM. Cadet and Parmentier declared that it contained no metallic or mineral substance, and that it was a vinous infusion of some bitter plant or plants. Alyon asserted that it was prepared with Gratiola; Mr. Moore that it was a vinous infusion of white hellebore with laudanum; however, Mr. Want that it was a vinous infusion of colchicum. Although most writers have adopted

Mr. Want's opinion, we should bear in mind that the proofs hitherto offered of its correctness, viz., analogy of effect, cannot be admitted to be conclusive, as is well shown by the fact that they have been advanced in favour of the identity of other medicines with the *Eau Medicinale*.

The power of colchicum to alleviate a paroxysm of gout is admitted by all; but considerable difference of opinion exists as to the extent of this power, and the propriety of employing it. Sir Everard Home, from observation of its effects on his own person, regarded it as a specific in gout, and from experiments on animals concluded that its beneficial effects in this malady are produced through the circulation.

Dr. Paris' observes: "As a *specific* in gout its efficacy has been fully ascertained; it allays pain, and cuts short the paroxysm. It has also a decided action upon the arterial system, which it would appear to control through the medium of the nerves." But if by the word specific is meant a, medicine infallibly, and on all patients, producing given salutary effects, and acting by some unknown power on the disease, without being directed by indications, undoubtedly colchicum is no specific for gout.

That colchicum alleviates a paroxysm of gout, I have before mentioned; but that alleviation is palliative, not curative. It has no tendency to prevent a speedy recurrence of the attack; nay, according to Sir Charles Scudamore, it renders the disposition to the disease much stronger in the system. Furthermore, by repetition its power over gouty paroxysms becomes diminished.

The *modus medendi* of colchicum in gout is an interesting, though not very satisfactory part of our inquiry. I have already stated that some regard this remedy as a specific; that is, as operating by some unknown influence. Others, however, and with more propriety, refer its therapeutical uses to its known physiological effects. "Colchicum," says Dr. Barlow, "purges, abates pain, and lowers the pulse. These effects are accounted for by assigning to it a cathartic and sedative operation; and it is this combination, perhaps, to which its peculiar virtues are to be ascribed." The fact that a combination of a drastic and a narcotic (as elaterium and opium, mentioned by Dr. Sutton, and white hellebore and. laudanum, recommended by Mr. Moore)" has been found to give, in several cases of gout, marked and speedy relief, seems to me to confirm Dr. Barlow's opinion. The idea entertained by Chelius, and adopted by Dr. G. Hume Weatherhead, that colchicum relieves gout by augmenting the quantity of uric acid in the urine, is not supported *by* fact, as I have already mentioned whether it acts by preventing the formation of uric acid in the system, I am not prepared to say.

In acute gout occurring in plethoric habits, blood-letting should precede the use of colchicum. This medicine should then be exhibited in full doses, so as to produce a copious evacuation by the bowels, and then the quantity must be considerably diminished. Though purging is not essential to the therapeutical influence of colchicum, it is admitted by most that, in a large number of cases at least, it promotes the alleviation of the symptoms. Hence, many practitioners recommend its combination with saline purgatives, as the sulphate of magnesia. Sir Charles Scudamore has experienced "the most remarkable success from a draught composed of *Magnesiae* 15 to 20 grains *; Magnes. Sulphat.* one to two drachm*; Aceti Colchici* one to two drachm; with any distilled water the most agreeable, and sweetened with any pleasant syrup, or with 15 or 20 grains of Extract. Glycyrrhiz."

2. In, rheumatism.– The analogy existing between gout and rheumatism has led to the trial of the same remedies in both diseases. But its therapeutical powers in the latter disease are much less marked than in the former. Rheumatism may affect the fibrous tissues of the joints, the synovial membrane, the muscles or their aponeurotic coverings, the periosteum, or the neurilemma, constituting thus five forms of the disease, which may be denominated respectively the *fibrous* or *ligamentous;* the *synovial, arthritic,* or *capsular;* the *muscular;* the *periosteal;* and the *neuralgic* forms of rheumatism. Of these, colchicum is said to produce its best effects in the synovial form. It is remarkable, however, that in all the severe cases of this variety of rheumatism which have fallen under my notice, the disease has proceeded unchecked, or was scarcely relieved by the use of colchicum. In one instance, that of my much lamented friend, the late Dr. Cummin (whose case is noticed by Dr. Macleod, in the *Lond. Med Gaz.* xxi. 858), the disease proved fatal by metastasis to the brain. In another melancholy, but not fatal case, the gentleman lost the sight of both his eyes, and has both knee-joints rendered stiff. In neither of these eases was colchicum of the slightest avail.

Of the mode of administering colchicum in "rheumatic gout," recommended by Mr. Wigan, I have no experience. He gives eight grains of the powder in some mild diluent every hour until active vomiting, profuse purging, or abundant perspiration take place; or, at least, till the stomach can bear no more. The usual quantity is eight or ten doses; but, while some take fourteen, others can bear only five. Though the pain ceases, the more active effects of the colchicum do not take place for some hours after the last dose. Thus administered, Mr. Wigan declares colchicum "the most easily managed, the most universally applicable, the safest, and the most certain specific in the whole compass of our opulent Pharmacopeia"but its use in these large doses requires to be carefully watched.

3. *In dropsy.–* Colchicum was used in dropsy with success by Storck. It has been employed in dropsical cases with the twofold view of purging and promoting the action of the kidneys. Given in combination with saline purgatives, I have found it beneficial in some cases of anasarca of old persons.

4. *In inflammatory diseases generally.–* Colehicum was recommended as a sedative in inflammatory diseases in general by the late Mr. C. T. Haden. He used it as an auxiliary to blood-letting, for the purpose of controlling arterial action; and gave it in the form of powder, in doses of six or seven grains, three or four times daily, in combination with purgatives, in inflammatory affections of the lungs and their membranes, and of the breasts and nipples. In chronic bronchitis it has also been found useful by Dr. Hastings.

5. *In fevers.–* The late Mr. Haden, and more recently Dr. Lewis, have spoken favourably of the use of colchicum in fever. In my opinion, it is only admissible in those forms of the disease requiring

an active antiphlogistic treatment. In such it may be useful as an auxiliary to blood-letting and cathartics.

6. *In various other diseases.–For expelling tapeworms,* colehicum has been found efficacious by Chisholm and Baumbach. *In some chronic affections of the nervous system* as chorea, hypochondriasis, hysteria, &c., Mr. Raven employed it with advantage. *In humoral asthma, and other chronic bronchial affections,* I have found it of great service, especially when these complaints were accompanied by anasarcous swellings.

Administration.– The cormi and seeds of meadow saffron have been employed in substance, in a liquid form, and in the state of extract.

Bruce A. Evans, M.D.

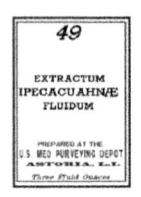

Extractum Ipecacuanhæ (Fluid extract of Ipecac) - Brownish liquid

In small doses (½ — 2 grains), it is used as a stimulant which is felt to benefit the stomach, exciting appetite and facilitating digestion. It is also used for producing beneficial expectoration and nausea in asthma, whooping cough, and in hemorrhage. Larger doses are emetic, and useful in narcotic poisoning.

Modern Perspective:

Ipecac is an effective emetic and, as most parents know, still in use for inducing vomiting after ingestion of certain poisonous but non-corrosive substances.

To the extent that ipecac was given in smaller, non-emetic doses or emesis was induced with larger doses as a means of "counter-irritation" or "revulsion" to treat inflammatory disease elsewhere, or to clean the bowels of postulated retained and toxic substances in dysentery, its use is counterproductive and ineffective according to current knowledge.

Period Reference:

The Elements of Materia Medica and Therapeutics – Jonathan Pereira, M.D. (Blanchard and Lee, Philadelphia, 1852) on the uses and administration of:
Ipecacuanha

Uses.– Ipecacuanha is employed in full doses as an emetic, or in smaller doses as an expectorant and nauseant.

1. *In full doses, as an emetic.–* The mildness of its operation adapts ipecacuanha for the use of delicate and debilitated persons, where our object is merely to evacuate the contents of the stomach. Thus, it is well fitted for the disorders of children requiring the use of emetics (as when the stomach is overloaded with food in hooping-cough, croup, &c.), on account of the mildness and certainty of its action. It is also exceedingly useful for adults (especially delicate females); thus, in gastric disorders, to evacuate undigested acrid matters from the stomach – to promote the passage of biliary calculi – as a counter-irritant at the commencement of fevers – in many inflammatory diseases (as acute mucous catarrh, cynanche, hernia humoralis, and ophthalmia) – in asthma – and as an evacuant in cases of narcotic poisoning. When the indication is to excite gentle vomiting in very weak and debilitated frames, Dr. Pye has shown that it may be effected. frequently with the utmost ease and safety by ipecacuanha in doses of from two to four grains. Dr. Cullen has expressed some doubt with respect to the correctness of this statement; but it is well known that ten grains of Dover's powder (containimg one grain of ipecacuanha) not unfrequently cause vomiting.

The mildness of its operation is not the only ground for preferring ipecacuanha to other emetic substances. Its specific power over the pulmonary organs and the stomach leads us to prefer it in maladies of these parts, in which vomiting is likely to be beneficial; especially in those affections in which the nerves appear to be more than ordinarily involved, as spasmodic asthma and hooping-cough. In the first of these complaints, Dr. Akenside has shown that it proves equally serviceable even when it fails to occasion vomiting, and merely produces nausea. He gave a scruple, in the paroxysm, to create vomiting, and, in the interval, five grains every morning, or ten grains every morning. Dr. Wright recommends gentle emetics of ipecacuanha at the commencement of the treatment of dysentery.

2. *In small doses, as a nauseant, antispasmodic, diaphoretic, and expectorant.–* When given in doses insufficient to occasion vomiting,

ipecacuanha is serviceable in several classes of complaints, especially those of the chest and alimentary canal.

a. In affections of the respiratory organs.– Nauseating doses of ipecacuanha are used with considerable advantage in acute cases of *mucous catarrh*. They favour expectoration and relaxation of the cutaneous vessels. In milder and more chronic forms, smaller doses, which do not occasion nausea, will be sufficient. In children, who bear vomiting much better than adults, full nauseating or even emetic doses are to be preferred.

" When a child becomes hoarse, and begins to cough," says Dr. Cheyne, " let every kind of stimulating food be withdrawn; let him be confined to an apartment of agreeable warmth; have a tepid bath; and take a drachm of the following mix- ture every hour, or every two hours if it produces sickness: Rx. Vini Ipecacuanhae 3 drachms; Syrupi Tolut. 5 drachms; Mucil. Acacia one fluid ounce. Mix.; and all danger will probably be averted; whereas, if no change be made in the quality of the food, and if he be sent into the open air, he will probably undergo an attack of bronchitis or croup."

In *hooping-cough,* in which disease considerable benefit is obtained by the use of emetic substances, ipecacuanha is frequently administered with advantage. After giving it to create vomiting, it should be administered in nauseating doses. In *asthma,* benefit is obtained by it, not only when given so as to occasion nausea and vomiting, as above noticed, but also in small and repeated doses. in both this and the preceding disease, the benefit procured by the use of ipccacuanha arises, not from the mere expectorating and nauseating operation alone of this remedy, but from its influence otherwise over the eighth pair of nerves. In *bronchial hemorrhage* (haemoptysis) the efficacy of ipecacuanha has been greatly commended. A. N. Aasheim, a Danish physician, gave it in doses of one-fourth of a grain every three hours during the day, and every four hours during the night. In this way it excites nausea, and sometimes even vomiting. It checks the hemorrhage, alleviates the cough, and relaxes the skin.

b. In affections of the alimentary canal – In *indigestion,* Daubenton gave it in doses just sufficient to excite a slight sensation of vermicular motion of the stomach, without carrying it to the point of nausea. Eberle tried it, in his own case, with evident advantage. An anti-emetic quality has been assigned to it by Schonheider. In *dysentery,* ipecaeuanha has gained no trifling celebrity, whence its name of *radix antidysenterica.* In severe forms of the disease no one, I suspect, now would think of relying on it as his principal remedy; but, as an auxiliary, its efficacy is not to be denied. The advocates for its use, however, are not agreed as to the best mode of using it. Sir George Baker and Dr. Cullen consider it to be of most benefit where it acts as a purgative; but this can scarcely be its *methodus medendi.* From my own observations of its use in the milder forms of dysentery met with in this country, I am disposed to ascribe its efficacy in part to its diaphoretic powers, since I have always seen it promoted by conjoining a diaphoretic regimen. But its tendency to produce an antiperistaltic movement of the intestines doubtless contributes to its antidysenteric property. It is best given, I think, in conjunction with opium. Its determination to the skin should be promoted by warm clothing, and the free use of mild, tepid aliment. Mr. Twining gave ipecacuanha in large doses (grs. six), with extract of gentian, without causing vomiting. Mr. Playfair recommends from half a drachm to a drachm of ipecacuanha, with from thirty to sixty drops of laudanum, to be given at the commencement of the disease.

c. In various other maladies.– As a sudorific, ipecaeuanha is given in combina- tion with opium (see *Pulvis Ipecacnanha: compositus)* in various diseases. On the continent it is esteemed as an antispasmodic. In uterine hemorrhage, also, it has been employed. In chronic visceral enlargements it has been administered as a resolvent.

Administration.– The usual dose of ipecacuanha, in *powder,* as an *emetic,* is grs. 15. But a much smaller quantity (for example, six, or four, or even two grains) will frequently suffice, as I have before mentioned. But a scruple, or half a drachm, may be taken with perfect safety. A commonly-used emetic consists of one grain of emetic tartar, and ten or fifteen grains of ipeeacuanha. For infants, half a grain or a grain of this root is usually sufficient to occasion vomiting. In all cases the operation of the remedy should be assisted by diluents. As a *nanseant*, the dose is from one to three grains. As an *expectorant* and *sudorific,* the dose should not exceed one grain; for infants, one-quarter or one-eighth of a grain. *Ipecacuanha, lozenges* contain usually from a quarter to half a grain of the powder, and may be used in catarrhal affections to promote expectoration. *Infusion of ipecacuanha* (prepared by digesting 2 drachms of the coarsely-powdered root in 6 fluidounces of boilingwater) may be used as an emetic, in cases of narcotic poisoning, in doses of one to two fluidounces.

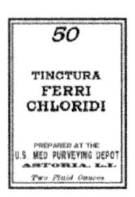

Tinctura Ferri Chloridi (Ferric Chloride; tincture of muriate of iron) -
Reddish-brown or yellow liquid

This is used as a tonic in debilitated patients or in low or aesthenic diseases. Tonics, as opposed to stimulants - which are used acutely to counter collapse - are used in the chronic phase of recovery to promote strengthening and recover, often in combination with an appropriate restorative diet. This tonic is given as 10-20 minims in water 2-3 times per day, increasing to 1-2 fluidrachms. It raises the pulse and promotes circulation. It is especially useful in erysipelas.

Modern Perspective:

Used as a tonic, this salt is a poor source of iron for anemia due to its highly acidic nature and corrosive properties. Ferric chloride solutions in water are used to etch circuit boards or precipitate impurities from water.

Some of the observed effects on the pulse and respiration may be due to the acidosis that can be induced by its ingestion. High doses, never achieved with this preparation, may also cause corrosive damage to the GI tract leading to pain, vomiting, and occasionally shock and death.

From a modern perspective, this is an ineffectual preparation.

Period Reference:

Bruce A. Evans, M.D.

The Elements of Materia Medica and Therapeutics – Jonathan Pereira, M.D. (Blanchard and Lee, Philadelphia, 1852) on the uses and administration of:

Ferric Chloride

Physiological Effects.– Tincture of sesquichloride of iron is, in its local action, one of the most powerful of the preparations of iron. It acts as an energetic astringent and styptic, and in large doses as an irritant. The large quantity of free hydrochloric acid which the tincture of the shops frequently contains, contributes to increase its irritant properties; and in Dr. Christison's *Treatise on Poisons* is a brief notice of a case in which an ounce and a half of this tincture was swallowed, and death occurred. in about six weeks – the symptoms during life, and. the appearances after death, being those indicative of inflammation of the alimentary canal. When swallowed in large medicinal doses it readily disorders the stomach. The general or constitutional effects of this preparation agree with those of other ferruginous compounds. It appears to possess, in addition, powerfully diuretic properties. Indeed, it would. seem to exercise some specific influence over the whole of the urinary apparatus; for, on no other supposition can we explain the remarkable effects which it sometimes produces in affections of the kidneys, bladder, urethra, and even the prostate gland. It colours the feces black, and usually constipates the bowels.

Uses.– It is sometimes, though not frequently, used as a topical agent. Thus it is applied as a *caustic* to venereal warts, and to spongy granulations. As an *astringent* it is sometimes employed as a local application to ulcers attended with a copious discharge; or as a *styptic to* stop hemorrhage from numerous small vessels.

Internally it may be employed as a *tonic* in any of the cases in which the other ferruginous compounds are administered, and. which I have already mentioned. It has been especially commended in scrofula.

In various affections of the urino-genital organs it is frequently used with great success. Thus, in retention of urine, arising from spasmodic stricture, its effects are sometimes beneficial. It should. be given in doses of ten minims every ten minutes until benefit is obtained, which frequently does not take place until nausea is excited. It has been used. with success in this malady by Mr. Cline, by Mr. Collins, by Drs. Thomas, Eberle, and Francis, and by Dr. Davy; However, Mr. Lawrence, alluding to Mr. Cline's recommendation of it, observes, " I believe general experience has not led others to place any very great confidence in the use of this remedy." In gleet and leucorrhoea it is sometimes serviceable. I have found it occasionally successful, when given in conjunction with the tincture of cantharides, in the latter stage of gonorrhea, after a variety of other remedies had failed. In passive hemorrhage from the kidneys, uterus, and bladder, it is likewise employed with benefit.

Administration.– The dose of it is from ten to thirty minims, gradually increased to one or two drachms, and taken in some mild diluent.

Bruce A. Evans, M.D.

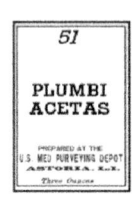

```
   51
PLUMBI
ACETAS
PREPARED AT THE
U.S. MED PURVEYING DEPOT
ASTORIA, L.I.
Three Ounces
```

Plumbi Acetas (lead acetate, sugar of lead) - Grayish powder

This substance is used as a powerful astringent in a dose of 1-3 grains in pill form every 2-3 hours. It is appropriate for hemorrhages from the lungs, intestines, and uterus. It is occasionally used for diarrhea or dysentery, most especially for typhoid with intestinal ulceration. It can be used for leucorrhea, given in a viscous solution with a penis syringe. Oral use may stain the mouth black after a time.

Note that lead poisoning is dangerous and must be watched for with any substantial or - use. Toxic symptoms of lead include, progressively:

- prodrome: lead/blue or slate/blue line on gum margins, especially incisors; bluish-red tint to gums; teeth stained brown, especially lowers; peculiar taste and breath odor; skin and sclera 'earthy-yellow' hue
- lead colic (severe, cramping abdominal pain)
- arthralgias (joint pains)
- paralysis of arms, legs
- disease of encephalon (encephalopathy, delirium, coma)

Modern Perspective:

The observation that lead acetate tended to dry weeping skin lesions led to its internal use for conditions associated with fluid discharges from tissues and, especially mucous membranes such as the Gastro-intestinal tract and the urethra.

While the substance does have a drying effect, and was used in paints and varnishes for just that reason, its well-known severe toxicity has ended that use. There is no beneficial effect on diseased tissues internally, whether or not the disease is associated with some sort of fluid discharge.

The toxicity acutely occurs with doses of 30 grams or more, and is associated with abdominal pain, stomach upset, cramps, tingling, and finally coma and death. Given in smaller doses over time - which was frequently done with chronic dysentery patients during the war - the cumulative dose would cause constipation, abdominal pain, and loss of appetite; or joint pain and sudden weakness (especially of the muscles that lift the hand) due to nerve damage. These symptoms were known to the medical profession during the war, and continuous administration of the drug was cautioned against.

Period Reference:

The Elements of Materia Medica and Therapeutics – Jonathan Pereira, M.D. (Blanchard and Lee, Philadelphia, 1852) on the uses and administration of:
Lead Acetate

Uses– Acetate of lead is administered *internally* to diminish the diameter of the capillary vessels, and lessen circulation, secretion, and exhalation.

Thus, we employ it in profuse discharges from the mucous membranes; as from the lungs, alimentary canal, and even the urino-genital membrane, In the mild cholera, so common in this country towards the end of summer, I have found acetate of lead in combination with opium most efficacious where the chalk mixture failed. I have used this combination in a few cases of malignant cholera, and in one or two with apparent benefit. In colliquative diarrhoea and chronic dysentery it occasionally proves serviceable. In phthisis it has been found beneficial, but only as a palliative; namely, to lessen the expectoration, check the night-sweats, or stop the harassing diarrhoea. Dr. Latham' speaks most favourably of the use of sugar of lead and opium in checking purulent or semi-purulent expectoration. I have repeatedly seen it diminish expectoration, but I have generally found it fail in relieving the night-sweats, though Fouquier supposed it to possess a specific power of checking them: they are more frequently benefited by diluted sulphuric acid.

In sanguineous exhalations from the mucous membranes, as epistaxis, hemoptysis, and hematemesis, and in uterine hemorrhage, it is employed with the view of diminishing the calibre of the bleeding vessels, and thereby of stopping the discharge: and experience has fully established its utility. It may be employed, in both the active and passive states of hemorrhage. It is usually given in combination with opium.

In bronchitis, with profuse secretion, it proves exceedingly valuable. It has been employed also as a remedy for mercurial salivation. It has been applied for this affection in the form of gargle by Soromd. Unless care be taken to wash the mouth carefully after its use, it is apt to blacken the teeth. On the same principles that we administer it to check excessive mucous discharges, it has been employed to lessen the secretion of pus in extensive abscesses attended with hectic fever.

There are some other cases in which experience has shown acetate of lead is occasionally serviceable, but in which we see no necessary connection between its obvious effects on the body and its remedial powers; as in epilepsy, chorea, intermittents, &c.

As a *topical remedy, we* use acetate of lead as a sedative, astringent, and desiccant. An aqueous solution of it is applied. to infirmed parts, or to secreting surfaces, to diminish profuse discharges. Thus, we use it in phlegmonous inflammation, in ophthalmia, in ulcers with profuse discharges, in gonorrhoea, and gleet. In the sloughing and ulceration of the cornea which attend purulent and pustular ophthalmia, its use should be prohibited, as it forms a white compound which is deposited on the ulcer, to which it adheres tenaciously, and in the healing becomes permanently and indelibly imbedded in the structure of the cornea. The appearance produced by this cause cannot be mistaken: its chalky impervious opacity distinguishes it from the pearly semi-transparent structure of even the densest opacity produced by common ulceration. The white compound consists of oxide (acetate?) of lead, animal matter, much carbonate of lead, traces of phosphate and chloride of the same metal.

A solution of acetate of lead may be employed as a disinfectant instead of the nitrate (see *ante,* p. 707).

Administration - Acetate of lead may be administered internally in doses of one or two grams to eight or ten grains, repeated twice or thrice daily, Dr. A. T. Thomson advised its exhibition in diluted distilled vinegar, to prevent its change into carbonate, which renders it more apt to occasion colic. It is usually exhibited in the form of pill, frequently in combination with opium. Acetate of lead and opium react chemically on each other, and produce acetate of morphia and meconate, with a little sulphate of lead. Experience, however, has fully established the therapeutic value of the combination. Sulphuric acid (as in infusion of roses), sulphates (as of magnesia, and soda, and alum), phosphates and carbonates, should be prohibited. Sulphuric acid, the sulphates, and phosphates, render it inert: the carbonates facilitate *the* production of colic pictonum. Common (especially spring) water, which contains sulphates, carbonates, and chlorides, is incompatible with this salt. The liquor ammoniae acetatis is incompatible with it on account of the carbonic acid usually diffused through this solution.

Bruce A. Evans, M.D.

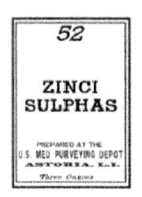

Zinci Sulphatus (zinc sulphate; white vitriol) -
Colorless transparent salt

The main use of this substance is as an external astringent or styptic to bleeding surfaces. It may be mixed with lard or simple cerate to form an astringent (drying and tightening) ointment for weeping surfaces.

Modern Perspective:

This substance, applied externally, does have a drying effect and a styptic effect on small vessel or capillary bleeding; however, unlike tannic acid, alum, and ferric subsulfate it causes significant local irritation and corrosion.

Period Reference:

The Elements of Materia Medica and Therapeutics – Jonathan Pereira, M.D. (Blanchard and Lee, Philadelphia, 1852) on the uses and administration of:
Zinc Sulphate

Uses.– As an *emetic* it is almost exclusively employed in poisoning, especially by narcotics. In these cases it is the best evacuant we can administer, on account of its prompt action. As an *internal astringent* it is administered in chronic dysentery and diarrhea, in chronic bronchial affections attended with profuse secretion, and in gleet and leucorrhoea. In the latter cases it is usually associated with terebinthinate medicines, and. is sometimes decidedly beneficial. As an *antispasmodic* it has been employed with occasional success in epilepsy, chorea, hysteria, spasmodic asthma, and hooping-cough. I have little faith in its efficacy in any of these cases. It has recently been spoken favourably of by Dr. Rabington in the treatment of epilepsy. He has sometimes given as much as thirty-six grains three times a day. As a *tonic* it has been serviceable in agues, but it is far inferior to sulphate of quina or arsenious acid.

As a *topical astringent* sulphate of zinc is most extensively employed. We use its aqueous solution as a collyrium in chronic ophthalmia, as a wash for ulcers attended. with profuse discharge, or with loose flabby granulations; as a gargle in ulcerations of the mouth, though I have found it for this purpose much inferior to a solution of sulphate of copper; as a lotion for chronic skin diseases; and as an injection in gleet and leucorrhoea.

Administration.– As an *emetic* the dose should. be from ten to twenty grains; as a *tonic, antispasmodic,* or *expectorant,* from one to five grains.

For external use, solutions are made of various strengths. Half a grain of the sulphate to an ounce of water is the weakest. The strongest I ever knew employed consisted of a drachm of sulphate dissolved in an ounce of water: it was used with success as an injection in gleet. But solutions of this strength must be applied with great caution, as they are dangerous.

Antidotes.– Promote the evacuation of the poison by demulcents. Afterwards allay hyperemesis by opium, bloodletting, and the usual antiphlogistic regimen. Vegetable astringents have been advised.

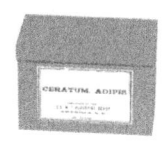

Ceratum

A simple, non-irritative salve to moisten and protect.

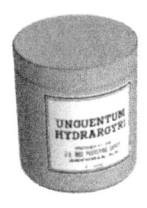

Unguentum Hydrargyri (mercury ointment; made of mercury, lard, suet) -   Bluish gray fatty substance

External form of mercury treatment, used either alone or in combination with internal treatment. It is useful in erysipelas, chilblains, and venereal buboes.

Modern Perspective:

Like most metals, elemental mercury does have antibacterial properties which may have given some benefit to the external use of this salve.
Most of the imagined benefits however (see calomel and mercury pills) have proven to be illusory.
This form, containing elemental mercury and used externally, is less toxic than calomel and provoked no systemic reaction.

Period Reference:

The Elements of Materia Medica and Therapeutics – Jonathan Pereira, M.D. (Blanchard and Lee, Philadelphia, 1852) on the uses and administration of:
Mercury Ointment

Physiologic Effects – Mercurial ointment possesses very little power of irritating the parts to which it is applied; but when either swallowed or rubbed into the integuments, it readily produces the constitutional effects of mercury. Thus Cullerier says, that three or four pills, containing each two grains of this ointment, and taken successively, have often sufficed. to excite violent salivation. He also tells us, that if the object be to produce ptyalism in a very short space of time, we may effect it by giving half a drachm of the ointment in the space of twenty-four hours.

When rubbed on the skin, it is capable of producing the before-mentioned constitutional effects of mercurials: and if the lard which it contains be not rancid, no obvious local effect is usually produced. Applied to ulcerated surfaces, mercurial ointment is a stimulant, and. in syphilitic sores is oftentimes a very useful and beneficial application.

Uses – It is rarely or never administered *internally* in this country, but has been much used on the continent, and with great success. Cullerier says, the difficulty with him has been rather to check than to excite salivation by it.

Applied *externally,* it is employed either as a local or constitutional remedy. Thus, as a *local* agent, it is used as a dressing to syphilitic sores, and is rubbed into tumours of various kinds (not those of a malignant nature, as cancer and fungus haematodes) with the view of causing their resolution. Sometimes, also, it is employed to destroy parasitic animals on the skin. As a *means of affecting the constitution* we use mercurial inunctions in syphilis, in inflammatory diseases, and, in fact, in all the cases (already noticed) in which our object is to set up the mercurial action in the system, more especially when the irritable condition of the digestive organs offers an objection to the internal employment of mercurial. It may be laid down as a general rule, that mercury may be used with more safety by the skin than by the stomach; but reasons of convenience, which I have already alluded. to, frequently lead us to prefer its internal use.

Administration - *Internally,* it is given in doses of from two to five grains, made into pills, with either soap or some mild powder, as liquorice. *Externally,* when the object is to excite very speedy salivation, half a drachm may be rubbed into the skin every hour, washing the part each time, and varying the seat of application. If, however, it be not, desirable or necessary to produce such a speedy effect, half a drachm, or a drachm, rubbed in night and morning, will be sufficient. During the whole course of inunction, the patient should wear the same drawers night and day.

When the friction is performed by a second person, the hand should be enveloped with soft oiled pig's bladder, turned inside out. Mercurial frictions ought not to be violent, but long continued, and, had better be.carried on near a fire, in order to promote the liquefaction and absorption of the ointment. In syphilis, and other diseases in which our sole object is the constitutional affection, it matters little to what part of the body the ointment is applied, provided the cuticle be thin (for this layer offers an impediment to absorption in proportion to its thickness). The internal parts of the thighs are usually, therefore, selected. However, in liver complaints, the inunctions are made in the region of the organ affected. The occasional use of the warm bath promotes absorption when the ointment is applied to the skin.

Appendix: Glossary of Period Medical Terms

acrid -
substance characterized by causing irritation of tissue surfaces to which it is applied

adjuvant -
a medication used in addition to the primary medication

adynamic -
an illness or phase of an illness characterized by features of a "low" disease, including prostration, wasting, and possible fatal issue through entrance into quiet confusion, somnolence, insensibility, and death

alterative -
an action of a therapeutic substance which changes the character of a body or tissue function, rather than simply stimulating or inhibiting the function

alvine -
having to do with the lower gastrointestinal tract

anasarca -
swelling caused by fluid accumulation of the limbs, the soft parts covering the abdomen and thorax, and even the face. Pitting of the skin results when an affected part is pressed with the finger, persisting after the finger is removed

anodyne -
substance having the action of relieving pain

anorexia -
suppression of the appetite

antiphlogisitic -
treatment or drug action designed to lower the excess tissue "excitement" characterizing the inflammatory or sthenic diseases

antiseptic -
drug action which prevents the mortification of tissues

antispasmodic -
treatment or drug action designed to suppress episodic nervous system action, as in epilepsy or chorea (uncontrolled extremity movements caused by nervous system disease)

apepsia -
inability to eat

apyrexic -
characterized by a lack of fever

Army -
A military force for self-contained active operations, made up of 2 or more infantry corps, cavalry regiments or division, and artillery, usually attached to the infantry corps. Commanded by a Lieutenant or Major General at the North, and a Full or Lieutenant General at the South.

articular extremity -
articular refers to the joint; the articular extremity is the end of a bone that participates in the formation of a joint

articulation -
joint or joint surface

asthenic -
category of disease characterized by lack of tissue excitement; associated with malaise, prostration, feeble and possibly slow pulse, and possibly progressing to a low delirium and death

astringent -
drug action which dries out wet surfaces such as ulcers, and tightens or contracts tissues.

Baron Larrey -
The chief surgeon of Napoleon's Grand Armee; a recognized expert and innovator in battlefield surgery

bid -
twice a day

bistoury -
formally, a French style of dissection knife. In North American practice, a knife with a straight or concave cutting edge, unlike the convex edge of the usual scalpel.

blennorrhea -
inordinate creation and discharge of mucous; when from the penis, gonorrhea

bougie -
a flexible cylinder, variable in size, to be introduced into the urethra, oesophagus, rectum, &c., for the purpose of dilating these (or other) canals, when contracted

Brigade -
The major tactical unit of an army, made up of 3-5 regiments which often share a common geographic or state origin. Usually commanded by a Brigadier General or, especially at the South, by a Colonel.

bronchocele -
an enlargement of the thyroid gland; common at the base of lofty mountains everywhere in the world. The enlargement may be massive. If the condition not be too chronic, iodine has great power over it and will generally cause its absorption.

bullae -
blisters, often filled with clear fluid

cachexia -
bodily wasting; a characteristic of low or asthenic diseases

calefacient -
substances which excite a degree of warmth in the part to which they are applied, as mustard, pepper, &c.

carminative -
medicines which relieve pain by causing the expulsion of flatus or gas from the lower gastrointestinal tract

cataplasm -
a medicine applied externally as a thick substance or pap, for instance to relieve pain, sooth, stimulate, irritate, etc.

cathartic -
drug action resulting in emptying of the lower gastrointestinal tract

caustic -
property of a substance that causes tissue damage, mortification, sloughing, and scarring on contact. Generally used to change the character of a skin or mucous membrane lesion for the better.

clyster -
an enema preparation to deliver medication to the patient

colliquative –
an epithet given to a discharge of fluid leading to rapid exhaustion

Comminuted -
Broken into a number of small pieces. A comminuted fracture is one in which rather than a clean break, the bone is crushed or broken into many small fragments in the fracture area.

congestive -
characterized by suffusion with excess blood

contiguity -
refers to resection of bone involving removal of a joint or part of a joint; i.e., a elbow resection or ankle disarticulation (removal of the foot by separating at the ankle joint)

continuity -
refers to resection of bone within the confines of one bone; amputation below a joint or resection of a piece of bone not involving a joint

contrastimulant -
procedure producing inflammation with the intention of drawing inflammation away from diseased tissue, as in the use of chest wall blisters for pneumonia

Corps -
The largest constituent unit of an army, consisting of 3-5 separate divisions each made up of 10-25 regiments grouped into brigades. Usually commanded by a Major General at the North and by a Lieutenant or Major General at the South.

cortex -
the outside surface of a structure; i.e., the grey matter of the brain or the dense outside layer of bone

coryza -
upper respiratory congestion with nasal discharge and stuffiness; a "cold"

counter-irritant -
substance producing inflammation with the intention of drawing inflammation away from diseased tissue, as in the use of chest wall blisters for pneumonia

cups -
equipment used either to draw blood from surface cuts placed in the skin by scarification (wet cups) or drawing blood to the surface of intact skin (dry cups), both by vacuum action. Used as a local form of bleeding, in place of systemic bleeding (venesection) in antiphlogistic treatment.

dejecta -
excretory products

depletion -
action of a therapeutic program designed to reduce the excess "excitement" of inflamed tissues characteristic of the sthenic diseases

depraved -
characterized by poisoned, low, or putrid blood; associated with a prostrating low disease.

desquamation -
shedding of a skin layer

dessicant -
substances which remove water from tissues

diaphoretic -
drug action which results in increased perspiration

disarticulation -
removal of a limb or part of a limb, or removal of the bone only in a resection, by separating it at a joint; e.g., no bone is cut

disinfectant -
agents that are capable of destroying miasma with which the air, clothing, &c. may infected; and capable of removing any incipient or fully formed septic condition from the living body or any part or product of it.

diuretic -
drug action which results in increased urination

Divisions -
The largest constituent unit of an army corps, consisting of 3-5 separate brigades each made up of 3-5 regiments. Usually commanded by a Major General.

dropsy -
disease accompanied by the accumulation of fluid in the tissues; may affect the limbs, the lungs, the abdomen, the brain, or other tissues depending on the disease process.

drug effect causing decreased nervous action or decreased pulse and heart action

Dysentery -
Severe diarrhea associated with painful, cramping urge to defecate and the presence of mucous in the dejecta, often accompanied by bits of tissue.

dyspepsia -
abdominal discomfort following eating

Eclectic Medicine -
A medical sect based on the choosing, from the available medical treatments, those that seem to be the best supported. In that sense, every physician should be "eclectic"; in practice the sect rejects many modern treatments and tends towards therapeutic nihilism - no treatment.

Effervescing Draught-
A cooling drink for fevers combining powdered bicarbonate of soda (1 scruple) with a vegetable acid such as tartaric acid or citric acid (18 grains), or lemon juice (4 fluid ounces); drunk while effervescing immediately upon mixing in water.

embrocation -
fluid rubbed into skin, e.g. liniment

emetic -
drug action resulting in vomiting, occasionally violent

emollient -
drug which sooths and moisturizes tissue

endocarditis -
inflammation of the heart valves

epigastric -
the upper middle abdomen

eruption -
skin lesions or rash appearing in the course of a disease

escharotic -
drug which causes tissue destruction

exacerbation -
disease worsening

exhalation -
emission of vapor by a tissue surface

expectorant -
drug action resulting in increased coughing productive of sputum

exudate -
substance exuded from inflamed tissues; may be pus or clear fluid

farinaceous -
dietary component made up of cereal substance

flux -
diarrhea

fomentations -
application of clothes soaked in hot water or medicated decoction

Fowler's Solution -
A prepartation of arsenic, comprising a solution of arsenite of potash, containing arsenious acid. It is potent and potentially toxic. It has anti-intermittent activity.

friction -
rubbing a part of the surface of the body more or less forcibly, with a flannel, brush, or: ointments, liniments, tinctures (moist friction); a useful means for exciting action at the sink for a counter-irritant or revulsive purpose.

functional -
derangement of a body function not associated with anatomic or pathologic change.

furred tongue -
drying and roughening of the tongue noted in some disease states; felt by some to be a special indication for the use of mercurial

gleet -
ghonorrhea; characterized by a thick mucous discharge from the penis and pain upon urination.

granulation -
tissue forming in the base of a healing ulcer or other open wound, as an initial stage of the healing process

hemorrhagic -
characterized by bleeding

hepatic -
relating to the liver

high diet -
a diet composed extensively of meat based products, appropriate to support and build up the constitution afflicted by a low or putrid disease state, such as typhoid or wasting due to a suppurating wound

Homeopathy -
A sect based on two principles: 1) Treating disease with drugs that cause effects resembling the symptoms of that disease. 2) Using these drugs in extremely diluted form, said to enhance their effect. In practice, the medicines are essentially water and without effect (either good or bad).

humors -
liquid substances felt to be responsible for disease in Galenic theory by virtue of the presence of excess of one or more over the proportions usually present in the natural state

hydrogogue -
medicines which attract and thus remove water from the tissues

hydrotherapy -
A sect based on the treatment of disease through the use of various applications of water immersions. Like other sects, it emphasizes relief from the sometimes harsh effects of orthodox "heroic" medicine's purgatives, &c.

impression -
effect of a disease process, stimulus, drug or treatment on the tissues of the body

inflammation -
tissue reaction characterized by heat, swelling, redness, and pain

integument -
the outer covering; the skin

intermission -

period of absence of symptoms during an intermittent fever

issue -

flow of exudate from the tissues, drawing away or draining these inflammatory products

laxative -

drug action resulting in relieving constipation by inducing bowel movements liquefacient - a medication with the property of liquefying solid depositions

leucorrhea -

a more or less abundant discharge of a white, yellowish, or greenish mucus resulting from inflammation of the membrane lining the genital organs.

ligate -

to tie off a structure by fastening a piece of silk or wire around it. This usually refers to tying off a blood vessel; either the cut end in a traumatic or surgical wound, or the artery at a site above an uncontrollable hemorrhage may be ligated to stop bleeding.

ligature -

silk or wire tied around a bleeding blood vessel to control hemorrhage

low -

disease with the characteristics of the *asthenic* diseases, with a lack of bodily or tissue excitement

low delirium -

a state of relatively quiet insensibility in which the patient is prostrate, confused, and tends to mutter incomprehensibly and pick at the bedclothes with his fingers; a common state leading to death in the low or sthenic diseases; in contrast to an active and raving delirium

low diet -
a diet composed mainly of vegetable and cereal products, appropriate to treat a patient with a sthenic disease. The less nutritious nature of the diet is intended to reduce the excess tissue and vascular excitement accompanying these inflammatory diseases.

malaise -
tiredness, lassitude; a characteristic of low or asthenic diseases

Materia Medica -
The body of knowledge of the sources, production, effects, and use of the drugs and medications available to the modern physician.

miasma -
substance responsible for disease; especially felt to be generated from or associated with damp or swampy ground or decaying vegetable matter

morbid -
diseased or relating to disease

Mortification -
The softening, partial liquification, and sloughing of tissue. The onset of mortification in a wound indicates an deviation from the healing process and a turn for the worse leading to chronic non-healing, pus-discharging wounds or to prostration, pyemia, and death.

moxa -
medication delivered to the skin mixed with a substance which is slowly flammable, burning from the top slowly towards the skin, gradually increasing the heat to the skin as it burns.

muttering delirium -
a state of relatively quiet insensibility in which the patient is prostrate, confused, and tends to mutter incomprehensibly and pick at the bedclothes with his fingers; a common state leading to death in the low or sthenic diseases; in contrast to an active and raving delirium

organic -
derangement of function of an organ or tissue that is associated with pathologic or anatomic change.

orifice -
from the Latin for mouth; an opening of an organ or an opening caused by a wound

osseous -
having to do with bone

paroxysm -
a periodic exacerbation or fit of a disease

Pavilion -
A style of permanent hospital construction based on numerous individual huts or pavilions with room for 25-50 beds each, and supplied with an open, undivided interior and numerous windows and roof vents for maximal healthy ventilation.

peccant -
morbid, not healthy; especially applying to humours when erring in quality or quantity

periosteum -
a fibrous, white medium surrounding bone, which unites bone to its surrounding parts and as it assists bone in growth and healing its preservation is essential for these to occur.

petichiae -
tiny spots of discoloration of the skin caused by focal bleeding

phlegmasiae -
an older term for the sthenic diseases, characterized by an excess of tissue and vascular excitement. This excess is recognized by such characteristics as a high fever, forceful and rapid pulse, flushing of the face and redness of involved skin areas, up to a raving delirium.

phlogistic -
tending to increase the excitement of the tissue or system, including a more forceful and rapid pulse, flushing, &c.

photophobia -
painful intolerance of light in the eyes

phthisis -
a chronic disease, most often affecting the lungs, leading to wasting and eventual death; consumption

pleurodynia -
pain on attempted breathing caused by inflammation in the lining of the lungs

primary hemorrhage -
hemorrhage or bleeding due directly to and occurring at the time of an injury, such as bleeding from a gunshot wound due to laceration of an artery by the missile

prostration -
state of collapse with extreme weakness, malaise and fatigue

pseudomembrane -
false tissue formed by the coagulation of an inflammatory exudate; seen in the throat in diphtheria and in the colon in some severe dysenteries

ptyalism -
salivation; derived from the Greek root for mercury, as this represents one of its most obvious effects.

purgative -
a medicine which acts more powerfully on the bowels than a laxative, stimulating the muscular coat and exciting increased secretion from the mucous coat. From the Latin "to cleanse".

purpura -
discoloration of the skin caused by bleeding; larger than petechiae

Purveyor -
A military official charged with obtaining necessary materials from private sources using government funds and disbursing them as needed for the operations of the army.

pustules -
pus filled blisters

putrescent -
putrid, redolent of rotting matter

putrid -
an epithet for some diseases, in which the matters excreted and even the breath give off a smell of rotting matter; low or prostrating diseases in general, due to presumed "rottenness of the blood.

Pyemia -
A consequence of a mortifying wound, pneumonia, or other disease in which the patient dies rapidly following the onset of shaking chills and rapid descent into delirium and coma.

qid -
four times per day

Quartermaster -
Positions in the military with authority and responsibility for provision of the material needs of the army, including munitions, arms, food, shelter, mounts, clothing, and means of transport.

rales -
crackling sounds heard in the lungs when the ear of the examiner is placed on the chest or a stethoscope is used; often indicates areas of congestion is the lungs

raving delirium -
an abnormal mental state often characterizing the terminal period of a sthenic disease such as brain fever, during which the patient is agitated, restless, and speaking loudly or shouting but without sense

reaction -
The state of activity which follows the action on the nervous system of certain disease producing influences, and to some extent opposes them by increased vitality or excitement; or, the opposing change or recovery after excitation or depression caused by a disease agent, a drug, or a treatment.

refrigerant -
drug action resulting in cooling of the patient

Regiment -
The basic unit of the armies, nominally consisting of slightly over one thousand officers and men , although veteran units rarely approach that number due to losses. Raised as volunteer regiments from a common area by State governments, and commanded by a colonel.

Regular -
a term applied to members of the military service holding rank in the central governmental military structure and appointed by the

Federal or Confederate government, as opposed to volunteers appointed by their several state governments.

repellant -
medicines which when applied to a swollen part, cause the fluids swelling it to recede; examples include astringents, cold water, and ice

repurcussive -
repellant; medicines which when applied to a swollen part, cause the fluids swelling it to recede; examples include astringents, cold water, and ice

resolvant -
medicines with the action of relieving enlargement of internal organs; said to be a property of mercurial

restorative -
any substance which strengthens and gives tone, such as, for example, wine.

revulsion -
production of inflammation by action of medication or physical stimulus at a remote site from the site of pathologic inflammation, in order to draw the unnatural inflammation away from the diseased organ

rubefacient -
drug which causes irritation and redness when applied to the skin

Sanitary -
Referring to the science of disease prevention through careful attention to cleanliness of the individual soldier, his food and especially water supply through appropriate location of latrines and disposal of camp waste, and placement of camps to avoid known health threats of the landscape.

scarify -

to cause scarring by intentionally damaging the surface of the skin or a wound, such as an ulcer. Usually done, either with medicines or physical means, in a hope that the character of the surface will be improved by the resultant healing process.

scorbutic -

relating to scurvy

scrofula -

a state of the system characterized by indolent, glandular tumors, chiefly in the neck. These tumors often discharge pus slowly and chronically and are slow or impossible to heal, leading to ulcers or occasionally healing through extensive scars.

secondary hemorrhage -

bleeding due to late effects from a wound or a surgical procedure, often due to gradual erosion or sloughing of an artery wall by an inflammatory process, dislodgment or erosion of a clot, &c. A feared cause of delayed death after a gunshot wound or amputation.

sedative –

sedative -

a property of a substance causing local or systemic decrease in signs of tissue and vascular excitement. A physical example of a local effect is the application of cold water dressings to a gunshot wound. Systemic examples include medications which slow the frequency and force of the pulse.

sialagogue -

a substance promoting increased production of saliva; e.g. mercurial

sinapisms -
mustard plasters

sinks –
latrines

slough -
the mortification and shedding of tissue from a wound or other skin affliction, such as an ulcer, etc.

solvafacient -
a medicine with the property of dissolving solid accumulations

sordes -
concretions resembling sand seen on the teeth, gums, and tongue in some disease states

spicule -
a splinter, usually of bone, caused by trauma to the bone such as a missile wound. Such separated fragments will die and function as a foreign body in a wound causing chronic pus drainage and impeding healing until they are expelled naturally or removed.

Staff Surgeons -
A general term for surgeons not attached to regiments and performing supervisory or administrative functions. At the North, mainly drawn from regular army surgeons or the *Surgeons and Assistant Surgeons of Volunteers,* appointments to which depended on federal application and successful examination.

sthenic -
diseases characterized by an excess of organism and tissue excitement; often associated with fever, inflammation, flushing, and increased heart action

stimulant -
drug action directly stimulating nervous action

stomachie -
a medicine that gives tone to the stomach

strangury -
difficulty passing urine, which is expelled drop by drop, accompanied by painful expulsive efforts

stupes -
cloth or leather strips soaked in or covered with an irritative substance such as turpentine and applied to the skin as a counter-irritant

styptic -
drug action which causes coagulation of blood; used to control bleeding

sudorific -
drug action resulting in increased sweating

supportive -
therapeutic action

suppurant -
drug action resulting in tissue damage and pus formation

suppuration -
tissue reaction resulting in pus formation

sybala -
hard balls of stool expelled at some point in course of dysentery

sympathy -
transmission of tendency to irritation or inflammation via nervous connections between organs or tissues

syncope -
a faint

tenesmus -
painful involuntary expulsive efforts of the lower colon; characteristic of dysentery

Thomsonism -
A medical sect based on the exclusive use of various gentle herbal and natural remedies. Named after its founder, who is said to have lost a loved one to what he viewed as the excesses of orthodox "heroic" medical treatments.

tid -
three times per day

tinnitus -
ringing or buzzing in the ears; seen as a toxic effect of quinine or cinchona use

tonic -
substance supporting an increase in nervous or tissue action

tormia -
griping abdominal pains characteristic of dysentery

torpid -
characterized by a low level of energy, activity, or function

Trephination -
Removal of a disk of bone from the skull with a circular type of saw designed for the purpose allowing the bone to be removed without damage to the underlying coverings of the brain. Usually done to allow placement of an elevator to lift a depressed skull fracture relieving brain pressure.

typhous -
fever characterized by depressed vitality of the system, a low fever.

venesection -
therapeutic bleeding by opening a vein with a lancet

vesicants -
drug action resulting in tissue drying

vesicle tenesmus -
painful expulsive efforts of the urinary bladder resulting from inflammation

Volunteer -
a term applied to a member of the military service holding rank by virtue of appointment by a state government, whether or not the body of troops involved has been accepted for service by the Federal or Confederate Army.

Author's Afterword

The content of this book was repurposed from my earlier interactive computer program:

The Civil War Surgeon Version 2.0 ©2016
which is no longer available.

The rationale was to continue to provide the content to a wider audience and make it more portable for use by Civil War medical re-enactors and living historians, as well as those without computer access (if those latter folks still exist!)

Bruce A. Evans, M.D.

Printed in Great Britain
by Amazon